Dr Ross Walker is an eminent cardiologist with a passion for people and health.

He graduated from the University of New South Wales with Honours in 1979 and was awarded the FRACP in 1986. His special interests are advanced echocardiography and preventative cardiology. He is the author of the bestselling books *If I Eat Another Carrot I'll Go Crazy*, *What's Cookin' Doc* and *Highway to Health*, all concentrating on lifestyle issues and in particular diet, antioxidants and health.

Dr Walker lectures extensively throughout the world to medical and business groups. He often discusses health and stress in the Australian media and has a weekly radio program on Radio 6PR in Perth and 3AK in Melbourne, where he discusses preventative health issues.

LOSE WEIGHT, GAIN ENERGY & LIVE LONGER

BY OPTIMISING YOUR CELL HEALTH WITH

THE CELL FACTOR

DR ROSS WALKER

M.B., B.S. (HONS), F.R.A.C.P.

MACMILLAN
Pan Macmillan Australia

First published 2002 in Macmillan by Pan Macmillan Australia Pty Ltd
St Martins Tower, 31 Market Street, Sydney

Reprinted 2002 (twice), 2003 (three times)

National Library of Australia
Cataloguing-in-Publication data:

Walker, Ross G. T.
    The cell factor: lose weight, gain energy and live longer
by optimising your cell health.

    ISBN 0 7329 1157 5.

    1. Cells – Health aspects. 2. Weight loss. 3. Health.
    I. Title.

611.0181

Typeset in 12.5/15 Adobe Garamond by Midland Typesetters
Printed in Australia by McPherson's Printing Group

CONTENTS

To my dear friend, Father Bob Bruce

'Each progressive spirit is opposed by a thousand mediocre minds appointed to guard the past.'
Maurice Maeterlinck

Introduction: Could we be wrong?

First, when I say 'we', who am I talking about? I am referring to collective wisdom. I am referring to health authorities, doctors, politicians and other people in positions of influence such as big business leaders. Mind you, we could've been right all along, but I have a very strong—and, I believe, healthy—suspicion that we have been wrong. I'm not suggesting we've been wrong in every single matter, but I am very confident that we've been given far too much misinformation about all the aspects of how to live life to the fullest.

Of course, with what I'm about to say, I will be considered arrogant, deluded and, some will say, plain crazy. But if you think about it, anyone who disagrees with conservative wisdom is usually vilified in some way. What then makes me so sure we have been getting it wrong?

I believe the evidence is obvious. Look around. We're all getting fatter; we're all getting sicker; most people you know are constantly tired; and, of course, everyone's stressed out of their brains. This is despite the fact we're living in a society absolutely geared towards the conveniences that make our life more comfortable.

How did we get it so wrong?

Ten thousand years ago, when we were hunter–gatherers, we spent most of our time searching for food and water to survive. These days, it's all about 'ease of life'—food is no longer a necessity but one of our major pleasures. The only hunter–gathering we do is jump into our cars and drive to the local supermarket, select our food, take it home and consume it at our convenience. This food is often so processed and packaged, and bombarded with so many chemicals, that the true nutrient value, which was once richly present, has been replaced with empty calories.

In developed societies our foods are abundant in fat, refined sugars and, to a lesser extent, protein. We are all overfed with these calories while the rest of the world continues to starve. The interesting irony is that our calorie-rich, overfed bodies are underfed with the vital micronutrients, vitamins, minerals and trace metals because of the over-processing and de-naturalisation of most of our foods. We lack adequate levels of the vitamins, minerals and trace metals that allow the cells of our bodies to function normally.

Another major issue in our modern world is comfort. One of the perceived comforts of the many comforts we have come to expect and take for granted is that of technology now performing many of even the simplest tasks that 50 years ago were the total realm of the human being. For example, our push-button world of entertainment. We can sit comfortably in our chair enjoying the full gambit of visual and auditory stimulation with the press of a remote control button. If we don't particularly like the show or piece of music, we can change it with the flick of a switch. This does not even require us to move from our lounge chair.

Away from work, technology has certainly made our lives easier, more comfortable and much more convenient. But at work, advanced technology has markedly increased our life stresses. With improved tele-communications—internet, email, voicemail, teleconferencing—we are immediately accessible to all and sundry. Many people working in inter-national companies make overseas phone calls well into the small hours of the morning instead of getting vital rest. Businesses want instant answers to stay ahead of the competition. Keeping pace with ever-changing technology, multiskilling, upsizing and downsizing of companies, and the constantly shifting new directions all contribute to increased stress. No longer can we expect to offer long service to one company with a gold watch at the end of our tenure—many people will have two to three different careers, and possibly more, throughout their lifetime. If a mistake is made at any level in the business or professional world, there is now the increasing threat of litigation, which also magnifies the day-to-day stress of performing any or all of the tasks of your occupation.

The world of today is an ever-changing—at times exciting and at times extremely terrifying—place to live. There can be no argument, however, that there is no precedent for our modern lifestyle. We, therefore, cannot learn from history and, in reality, we do not know the long-term effects this new 'Information Age' will have on our health and general wellbeing.

Over the centuries, our medical system has evolved with its fascinating blend of art and science. In the less educated, less technology-based world of yesteryear, the medical profession was revered and respected. Doctors relied on caring, bedside manner and an interesting blend of magic and confusing medical terms to deliver a service that seldom cured, occasionally relieved, but generally comforted those afflicted. The doctors' services were greatly appreciated and, in reality, hope was the major ingredient.

With technology being such an important part of today's medical services, most people feel lost in the science. The old-world view of the medical profession as a caring, compassionate service no longer applies and most doctors are viewed as elite technocrats in a system that churns through patients with little regard for their deeper issues. The paternalism of yesteryear still persists, but often without the compassion.

One of the unfortunate ingrained remnants of the old medical system is the so-called 'disease model'. Basically, you visit a doctor with a symptom, which is your ticket into the system. The doctor forms an hypothesis from your cluster of symptoms and physical signs, often orders a series of expensive and usually unhelpful tests, followed by a diagnostic hypothesis and subsequent treatment program that usually involves drugs, surgery, or a combination of both.

In my field of cardiology, there are myriad treatments available for a number of different conditions affecting the vascular system. These include well over 50 drugs to treat high blood pressure, numerous cholesterol-lowering pills and a host of cardiologic interventions to treat blockages, electrical instability or valve problems. There are also a large number of surgical procedures that can be performed in many different fashions to restore people's hearts to good health. Or so we are led to believe.

The reality is that almost all of these drugs, interventions or surgical procedures at their best slow down the inevitable progression of the underlying condition. For example, the modern cholesterol-lowering pills used alone can only hope to slow the progression of fat build-up in the arteries. They certainly do not arrest this process, nor reverse it.

Because people in our society are obviously becoming fatter, sicker, more fatigued, more dissatisfied and more stressed, it is apparent to me that we have got it all wrong.

We are constantly being fed the 'no pain, no gain' message by health professionals (I prefer to call them 'the health police'), and the way to good health is a low-fat, high-carbohydrate diet with some exercise thrown in. When someone thinks of a lifestyle change they basically say, 'I'll change from butter to margarine', 'I'll switch from white to brown bread', or possibly, 'I'll have one less coffee per day'. These major life changes, of course, last for a few weeks and then, like most human beings, a person slips back to their old habits in the blink of an eye. This dietary collective wisdom we're being bombarded with year in, year out, is obviously not working.

When you turn to the cover of any popular magazine, each week there is a new wonder diet that will strip kilos from your stomach and hips; pulverise cellulite into the next dimension; and even improve your sex drive. If you believe this, you probably also believe in the tooth fairy and that many cigarette company executives still do not consider smoking addictive.

Not only do I believe we are getting the dietary messages wrong for reasons that will be explained later in the book, but I also believe the work environment has got it totally wrong with the corporate structure over the past 20 to 30 years, completely destroying the value of the individual and the greater good of society. Service to the customer and the employees has gone out the window and it is now basically analysis of the bottom-line profits.

With our pathetic dependency on petrochemicals to fuel our cars and our industries, we are destroying the earth and ourselves; but who cares, it's making a minority of extremely wealthy individuals even wealthier. For example, in the 1950s Los Angeles had one of the best public transport systems in the world. This was purchased by a major automobile company and subsequently closed down. A flight into Los Angeles airport or a drive along one of its major freeways will show you the result of this marvellous decision.

Let's not, however, just blame the petrochemical companies for our current lot; let's also look at many of the major food and drug companies that are flooding the market with myriad products that are, certainly, offering us short-term solutions, but are chronically poisoning our bodies. A simple principle I will develop through this book is: if it is in a box, a bottle, a tube or a packet, you can be fairly confident there are chemicals inside the container to ensure that the stuff can sit on a shelf for a few months at least.

If this is the case, have you ever wondered what these chemicals do once they get into your body? Of course, nothing has been proven in one of those marvellous 'controlled' clinical trials (usually sponsored by the company that makes the product). Therefore, this is enough justification to continue the practice! We live in a chemical world from the moment we switch on the air conditioning, soap ourselves in the shower, wash our hair, use deodorant, shave, or put on make-up (or whatever other means you use to make yourself more beautiful—or in some cases, less offensive to the people around you). We then shovel down our throats highly processed and packaged foods containing even more chemicals before venturing outside into an air that is usually polluted with thousands of major and minor chemicals.

Putting the chemical story aside for a moment, we are also poisoning ourselves with inactivity and stress. As I stated earlier, with the increasing comforts of our world we move less. And despite the fact that we live in a playful universe where almost everything happens with the minimal amount of stress as far as nature is concerned, we are constantly under pressure from external or internal forces.

The health police pick on saturated fat and refined sugar as the major cause for many health problems, especially in my field of cardiology. I must state strongly that I disagree with this and believe that our current health crisis is due to two major factors: chronic poisoning from many sources, and nutritional deficiency—both in our diet and at the cellular level.

How do we get it right?

For too long we have concentrated on the consequences and associations of particular diseases. For example, if someone is a cardiac patient and suffers cholesterol or high blood pressure, like many people they may make the rather bizarre statement, 'I've got cholesterol and it's clogged up my heart.'

We seem to want some sort of simplistic explanation for everything that happens. When it comes to our bodies, we are ignoring the simple fact that it is the *cell* where 'it' all takes place. We look at the end result—in this instance, the clogging of the arteries—as being one form of cardiovascular disease, such as a heart attack, stroke or sudden death, the same as we look at the development of a tumour as cancer. In doing so, we are missing the vital point.

Any major disease occurring in our body commences in a single cell. Rather than wait until cell after cell is affected by whatever process started it in the first place, we should be looking at the true reasons these conditions occur at the cellular level. This is the 'Cell Factor'.

The human body, and therefore the human cell, was not designed to live forever. It was definitely designed, however, to live in symbiosis with nature. In our modern, technology driven, chemically based society we have moved so far away from this natural internal and external environment, all manner of diseases are now occurring. Rather than blame these diseases on cholesterol, high blood pressure or stress, we should be taking them back to the root cause: the cell.

The two major factors in our modern society which are having such a profound effect on our cells are chronic poisoning from many different sources, and multiple nutritional deficiencies. All we need to do is look and ask around. Most of our friends, colleagues or people on the street are overweight, tired and many are looking very unhappy. Restore the health of your cells and you restore the health of your body.

The Cell Factor

For even the brightest mind, reading health books can be pretty dull. In fact, when an author becomes too technical it can be about as interesting as a graduation speech. I would still, however, like you to understand how a cell works so I can develop my theory of the Cell Factor.

Let me make the very strong analogy between a cell and a factory. In the factory, there is an entrance that faces the road. Trucks enter the factory from the road to the delivery area. The raw materials to be processed are delivered to the appropriate parts of the factory and the workers in the factory use various machines to manufacture particular products.

The factory, of course, needs a constant and reliable power supply. It also has strong, sturdy walls to protect against the weather and robbery. The management team headed by the boss work in separate offices in the factory so regular, consistent instructions can be given to the workers. The quality control section is also housed in the management offices. There is a health and safety surveillance team along with security to maintain the wellbeing of the workers and to ensure that the workers, the property and the products are safe. There is also a cleaning and maintenance team that ensures the factory is spotless and any waste products are transported out of the factory and taken to an area away from the factory for adequate disposal. The management team also has to organise the regular delivery of products to the factory. It is the job of the management team to ensure the factory has an adequate, though not excessive or depleted, supply of raw materials to ensure maximum efficiency within the factory.

There are many factories supplying similar and different goods. There is also integrated smooth communication between all the factories in one area and between all the areas of one region and between all the regions of one city and between all the cities of one country. It is quite amazing how man has borrowed so much from nature! The functioning of our community is exactly the same as the functioning of our bodies—down to the functioning of the unit; which is the cell.

The roads in the body are the blood vessels. The blood vessels deliver the products to the cells in the form of either macronutrients (i.e. fat, sugar and protein) or micronutrients (i.e. vitamins, minerals and trace metals). Without an adequate supply of all these products, the cells cannot function efficiently and some form of disease will soon ensue.

Oxygen is vital to all the cells of the body and this is delivered via the red cells in a protein known as haemoglobin. Oxygen enters the cell across the outer covering, known as the membrane, and travels into the energy-creating area known as the mitochondria. The mitochondria burns oxygen with the breakdown products of fat, sugar and, to a lesser extent, protein (the major fuels), creating the major energy-generator known as ATP. (Please bear with me; all this will become relevant.)

The cell wall (membrane) is made up of 75 per cent fat mainly in the form of phospholipid. This fat needs to be made up of healthy, natural fats and includes the essential fatty acids Omega-3 and Omega-6, as well as a significant amount of saturated fats and cholesterol. If the outer wall is not functioning properly, it is difficult for the nutrients (i.e. the delivery products) to enter the cell properly and nourish the cell. If the cell wall does not have normal amounts of these essential fatty acids then it cannot deliver adequate amounts of nutrients to all of the different areas of the cell for normal processing.

The liver has many functions and is the major factory in the body. If you removed someone's liver, they would be dead within 24 hours. The liver makes a whole series of proteins which carry nutrients and other substances around the body. Without albumin, a water-soluble protein, many of these substances are 'all dressed up with nowhere to go'. Not only does the liver make numerous proteins for anything from transport to blood coagulation, it is also a vital area for the clearing of substances through the bile. This is why many people, after a heavy night on the grog, feel extremely sick for a day or two—because the function of the liver is acutely affected and the by-products of the excessive amounts of alcohol have not as yet washed out of the body.

The function of a muscle is, of course, to move. There are a whole series of proteins made by the muscle cells which allow the muscle to contract and relax, depending on the needs of the body at that particular time. The production of all of these proteins requires a constant supply of amino acids (these are the breakdown products of proteins), some of which are made in the body and some of which we *must* get from our diet. Control of protein production and every other function of the cell, including cell division, occurs in the nucleus of the cell, which also controls its own DNA production and the timing of cell division.

Regardless of the cell involved, almost all of the cells in the body have their own control room known as the nucleus. This is where the management team works and without the nucleus, the cell cannot continue to perform all of its many functions.

Substances such as oxygen and carbon dioxide do not require assistance in diffusing in and out of cells. Carbon dioxide is, of course, the major by-product of energy production in the cell and must be taken up in the red cell that has lost oxygen and delivered back to the lungs where it is breathed out. Substances such as glucose require energy to enter the cell. Glucose latches on to a receptor, which is like a lock on the surface of the cell, and this receptor then delivers glucose to the cytoplasm, which is the factory floor.

The immune system, which is made up of different types of white cells and other chemicals made by these cells, basically acts as the security guard and health and safety officer of the cell, cleaning up the by-products and ensuring no foreign substances attack the cell. The white cells also function like any other cell in the body, making their own proteins and maintaining their own health.

Components of the white cells, known as T-cells and B-cells, are basically mobile nervous systems. These cells contain their own thought processes and contain an enormous amount of memory about many of the bugs that have plagued us over the centuries and they can also develop new killing mechanisms to destroy invading bacteria, viruses and other foreign substances. The T-cells produce chemicals that can destroy viruses and tumours, whereas the B-cells are more geared to producing antibodies. There are many other white cells that have numerous actions. Some of these white cells are for acute bacterial infections, whereas others are very much geared for dealing with allergies.

The major problem for the body is when synthetic fats and synthetic sugars are introduced into the system. A cell membrane cannot distinguish between synthetic fat and natural fat. When synthetic fat in the form of trans fatty acids is introduced, these trans fatty acids incorporate into the cell membrane instead of natural fats, deranging the membrane and making it hard and impermeable to nutrients. The inner part of the cell is now being starved of nutrients, therefore it cannot perform its function correctly. Thus, the cell lacks energy, and thus we lack energy. We feel fatigued because our cells are fatigued because they lack energy.

What is the most common, most acute source of energy? Some form of sugar. If our membranes become deranged and there is a lack of nutrients travelling into the cells, we need constant sugar fixes throughout the day in an attempt to overcome our chronic cellular malnutrition and we become carbohydrate junkies. Also, if the membrane is not working properly, the protein receptors, which sit on the cells and allow the entry of sugar, fat and protein into the cell, do not work properly.

The major doorman, which allows entry of sugar, and to a lessser extent, fat and protein, into the cells, is insulin. The body's response to this deranged membrane function is to make more insulin. The body then becomes resistant to the effects of insulin and the insulin level rises in the bloodstream. One of the major effects of excessive insulin is the laying down of fat. The more sugar we cannot get into the cell, the more insulin we make and the more weight we put on as the insulin rapidly deposits the sugar as fat into our fat cells.

You can see the pattern here: fatigue, carbohydrate craving, rise in

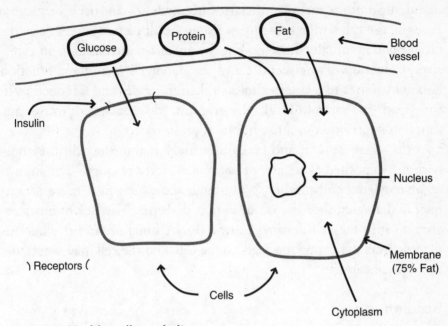

Figure A: Healthy cell metabolism

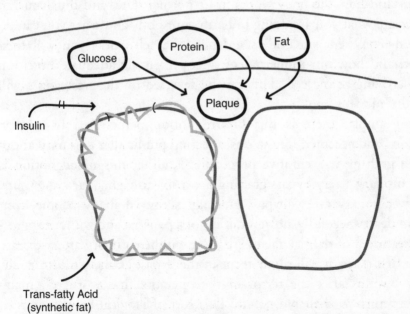

Figure B: Unhealthy cell damaged by synthetic fats leading to fatty, sugary, proteinaceous plaque formation

blood sugar from excessive dietary carbohydrates and lack of glucose entering the cell with a subsequent rise in insulin levels leads to obesity, fatigue and eventually diabetes. The insulin also contributes to an excessive production of triglycerides and the deranged membrane function also contributes to a rise in cholesterol triglycerides and a reduction in the good cholesterol, HDL. In additon, this deranged membrane function contributes to a rise in blood pressure.

As the sugar, protein and fat cannot make it into the cell, they now becomes deposited as sugary, proteinaceous fatty plaques—also known as 'glycosylated end products'. Although these are much more prominent in diabetics, they also occur in non-diabetics. The lack of nutrients arriving into the cell destroys normal DNA function and the nucleus then delivers the wrong messages to the cell, and the cell may eventually become cancerous.

Read on . . .

To understand why you get sick in the first place it's important to understand how the body works in its normal state, and thus you can appreciate what you are doing to harm your body and what you can do to heal it. When you understand how the cell works you will then understand how our modern society is preventing adequate nutrition from arriving at the cell. This can be reversed by the strategies I will introduce in this book.

For example, there is this bizarre notion perpetrated by cardiac surgeons and accepted by the unsuspecting public that coronary artery bypass grafting is a curative procedure. Another misguided notion is that coronary artery bypass grafting has a six- to eight-year *use-by date*. Firstly, coronary artery bypass grafting has saved many people from certain death. Secondly, however, it is not a panacea and without aggressive treatment of the risk factors that caused the coronary artery disease in the first place, it will surely recur in the bypass grafts. Unfortunately, a few months after the terror of the operation has worn off, many people return to their old habits. This sort of illogical behaviour is so typical of human beings. The further we are from a terrifying event, in many cases, the less impact it has on us.

It is my firm opinion, which I will reinforce throughout this book, that in almost all cases heart disease and many other potentially fatal or debilitating diseases can be stabilised and, in many cases, reversed. The earlier a diagnosis is made, the easier it is to reverse. Despite this, I have seen dramatic reversals of atherosclerosis (fatty plaque build-up) in people after bypass surgery. It really depends on how motivated you and your doctor are to achieve this end.

There is overwhelming evidence that common environmental poisons, such as diet, cigarette smoking and inactivity, contribute to atherosclerotic disease. For example, the relative risk of coronary heart disease for inactive people is twice as high as people who are active. The simple habit of enjoying one or two drinks of alcohol per day is associated with an across-the-board 30 to 40 per cent lower risk of coronary heart disease.

In a study known as the Oslo Trial, which combined dietary advice and anti-smoking advice, the reduction of saturated fat combined with an Omega-6 polyunsaturated fatty diet, along with a high-fibre diet and the cessation of smoking, led to around a 50 per cent reduction in fatal and non-fatal heart attack among people who received the dietary and anti-smoking advice compared with the control group that did not receive any advice.

But most diseases have multiple causes, including multiple genes and multiple environmental factors. In my opinion, genes probably contribute somewhere around 30 per cent to most illnesses; the other 70 per cent comes from the environment.

This is why I persist in supporting and promoting preventative health advice. This is why I became involved with CT scanners as a means to detecting risk factors before they become a problem. There are now numerous studies to show that coronary artery calcium scoring using CT scanning technology is the best non-invasive predictor for long-term, future cardiac events. Most of these studies show that a high calcium score is a 10 times better predictor for heart disease than high cholesterol.

BENEFITS OF CT SCANNERS

The calcium score is a software-created score derived from the area of the calcium detected in the arteries multiplied by a density factor. A score of zero is what we would all like, which implies no calcium and therefore very little fat in our arteries. As I will explain in the later section on atherosclerosis, calcium seen on a CT scan suggests atherosclerosis. A zero score on the CT scan certainly does not imply that there is absolutely no atherosclerosis, but all of the studies, however, do reinforce the fact that a zero score implies a very low risk. For example, a male of 50 with a zero score has a 0.1 per cent risk per year of some sort of cardiac event. Compare this to an average middle-age male, who's risk is around 1.0 per cent per year. Then compare this to someone with a score above 1000 who has a yearly risk of either a heart attack or sudden death of around 25 per cent per year.

Zero	very low risk
1–100	mild calcification, low risk
100–400	moderate calcification, moderate risk
greater than 400	high risk

I am more than happy to explore any alternative treatments and have personally derived great benefit from many of these treatments in maintaining my own health. For example, around five years ago I underwent a septoplasty because of a deviated septum (basically, a broken nose) I received from my years of playing rugby union. For around 20 years after I hung up my rugby boots and put on my soccer boots, I had to use nose drops just to be able to sleep at night because my nose was blocked from the deviated septum. I was sick of using inhaled steroid nasal spray, which in my case was not affording me much benefit. So I underwent an operation on my sinuses and septum, and had tremendous relief compared with the pre-operative situation. I was still, however, troubled by some degree of nasal congestion.

One night I was lecturing to a group of general practitioners and one of my colleagues said that he had obtained incredible relief for his sinuses from a herbal preparation that contained fenugreek and horse-radish and a number of other herbs. I dutifully started taking one of these herbal pills twice a day and have been doing so for the past three years with a stunning improvement in my degree of nasal congestion.

I must say that there is absolutely no evidence-based medicine to back up the claims of this herbal preparation, but I have since suggested this simple, harmless treatment to many of my patients and have universally seen a great response in what can be a very common debilitating and irritating condition.

This, however, is not particularly controversial and pales into insig-nificance when compared to the controversies occurring throughout the world in treatments for the more serious conditions such as heart disease and cancer.

This book is divided into two parts. The first outlines the risk factors for diseases, such as cardiovascular problems and cancer, and provides some treatment options. But more importantly it gives you the opportunity to evaluate your current health status and work out how you may prevent any medical condition from deteriorating. The second part is the healthy lifestyle program covering the five steps to optimum cellular health.

For those who have read my previous books, you will understand that there is always a strong numerical structure in what I write. This theme is the universal Rule of Five. Just look at nature. There are five digits on your hands and feet. There are five senses. There are even five seasons if you count Frankie Valli!

I believe all preventative medicine starts with the individual—you. You can read a book, such as this, finish it and say, 'Yes, that was interesting' . . . but do nothing about it. I challenge you to make the decision today to bring in some action into your life. If you truly follow the principles detailed in this book, I have no doubt you will restore your cells to good health. You will lose weight, develop an enormous source of energy and markedly reduce your risk for any manner of oncoming nasty diseases. Confucius once said 'A journey of a thousand miles begins with a single step'.

The first step in any new journey is to make the decision. If you make the decision today that you want to change, you want to lose weight, you want to feel more energy and you want to be healthier . . . you have just taken the first step.

PART I

Understanding Disease Risk Factors

Is it in the genes, or the jeans?

There is a wonderful saying that states: 'It is our genetics that load the gun but our environment that pulls the trigger.' There is no doubt that for most of us, this is true. Very occasionally we hear of a person in their eighties who has been a constant smoker and drinker, is overweight and still appears reasonably healthy. I must admit, I have seen the occasional person who smoked and drank and ate the wrong foods into their eighties but I cannot say I ever met anyone in this category who was particularly healthy. I believe there is always a price to pay for poor health habits—even if that price isn't a reduction in life span. Unfortunately, however, we hear too frequently of the opposite scenario.

Malcolm Sefton was 43 years old. He had never smoked, was a lifelong exerciser who had competed in marathons and numerous triathlons, was a very light drinker, and was very conscious of his diet. He didn't have an ounce of body fat. He woke regularly at 5.30 a.m. to run 5 kilometres before he went off to his job as a chartered accountant. One morning he didn't feel particularly well and had an uneasiness in his chest during the run. He returned home, showered, had breakfast, and then went to work feeling as if he was developing a virus. When he arrived home he didn't feel like eating and told his wife he was going to bed early. The next morning he woke at 5.30 a.m. still feeling unwell, but decided a run in the still morning air would make him feel better. Malcolm never returned home. The autopsy revealed extensive coronary artery disease with a fresh rupture of a fatty plaque leading to a fatal heart attack.

Although this story is tragic, it is relatively common. Malcolm was under the mistaken impression that because of his lifestyle, he was immune to major diseases. Unfortunately, what we would normally associate with heart disease accounts for only around 50 to 60 per cent of all coronary cases. Had Malcolm had a thorough check-up at a preventative screening centre, his condition would have almost certainly been detected early on and his death prevented.

So what is the genetic story? With the recent completion of the mapping of the human genome it has been suggested that human beings contain somewhere between 30 000 and 100 000 sets of genes. What most people don't realise is that genes not only determine your external bodily appearance, there are also genes that cater for every reaction in the body. Although these genes are fixed structures, the influence of the genes on our external appearance and internal metabolism or body functioning very much depends on how those genes are treated.

For example, identical twins have exactly the same DNA patterns. If you were to put one twin in a comfortable, happy life where the stresses are minimal and the other in a life where their body is constantly abused by external stress—the sun, alcohol and cigarettes, etc.—in almost all cases you will find the stressed twin looks anywhere between 10 and 15 years older than the happier twin. An abused body will cave in long before its time. Therefore, our genes cannot determine every aspect of our existence as there is a strong gene: environment interaction.

There is a set of genes that codes for stress. If I placed you under enormous stress for a few months, a set of genes will be switched on and your body will react by making your heart race, raising your blood pressure, elevating your blood sugar levels and depressing your immunity. It would probably take four to five weeks after the stressors have ceased for all of these processes to settle down—however long it takes the proteins created by the switched-on stress genes to break down through normal bodily processes. This is why it usually takes a few weeks of holidays before you are starting to feel 'human' again after a year of intense stress.

A GENE BREAK

Holidays are a vital way to recharge your batteries and fight against the stress genes that cause us so many problems. I often have people come into my practice and say, 'Doc, I haven't had a holiday in 10 years!' as if they are enormously proud of themselves. I say to them, 'Well, you're an idiot!' (I don't really make such an unsubtle comment—but I probably should!)

Another interesting aspect of the gene story is the mistaken belief that genes determine our life. If genes were the basic life forces, then cloning would certainly make us immortal. But human beings have been cloned since recorded history, in the form of identical twins. It would be ludicrous to suggest identical twins are the same person. Of course they have the same DNA, but there is definitely something different about each twin. Even Siamese twins, which are physically joined, have two separate entities within the joined body. One day, you may be able to clone another individual that has a seemingly identical genetic make-up to yourself, but you certainly wouldn't have the same feelings and emotions as the cloned person.

Another issue, which is not generally discussed, was demonstrated in the first cloned animal, Dolly the sheep. Dolly was cloned from a six-year-old adult female. Therefore Dolly's DNA was already six years old. A few years on, Dolly is ageing at a great rate and is significantly obese. Her DNA is breaking down. This strongly suggests that DNA ages with the rest of the body and it is important to consider the implications of this before reproductive cloning is even considered to be a reasonable scientific step. I am only discussing the science of cloning, not the more complex and difficult ethical issue.

I think you can see from this discussion that it is not just a matter of 'one gene determines one action' regardless of the environment; it is much more complex, as the expression of our genes can be altered by physical, emotional and psychological stressors and simply by ageing. Thus, anything from food, legal or illegal poisons, to a difficult work environment or a bad marriage can affect the way our genes behave. But, there still are much less common (though still very important) genetic diseases that, regardless of how well we look after ourselves, will cause us all sorts of bother.

The major fatal or debilitating diseases in people are cardiovascular disease and cancer. What causes these diseases to manifest in an individual are genetic and environmental factors. There is almost never just one particular cause. Now, I would like to discuss these diseases from both a genetic/scientific basis and an environmental cause/factor basis.

Chronic nutritional poisoning

What's the first piece of advice you would get from a doctor or nutritionist if you wanted to lose weight or had just suffered a heart attack? They'd probably say, 'Cut back on your fat intake.' Well, there is now great doubt about this long-perpetrated piece of pseudo-wisdom. Public health reasearchers in London published a review of the relationship between dietary fat intake and the prevention of heart disease in the *British Medical Journal* in March 2001. Their conclusion was that there is a small, but potentially important reduction in cardiac risk with the reduction or modification of dietary fat intake. This is especially noted in trials of greater than two years.

It's an interesting turn of phrase—'a small, but potentially important reduction'. When I looked carefully at this review, which analysed 27 studies involving the modification of dietary fat intake, I found the results quite fascinating. Firstly, and most importantly, alteration of dietary fat intake had no effect on total death rates; death from cardiac disease was only reduced by 9 per cent and cardiac events, such as sudden death or heart attack, were only reduced by 16 per cent. If these trials were followed for longer than two years, however, there was a

23

24 per cent protection from cardiac events, but again, no difference in total death rates from all diseases. So *why* is the health profession so strong on people changing their fat intake?

I believe the whole emphasis on fat has been in the wrong direction. In the chapter on cardiovascular disease, I introduce the concept of pattern A and pattern B cholesterol profiles. Pattern B is characterised by small, dense LDL cholesterol—the really nasty type of LDL, the one which is easily oxidised and finds it much easier to cross damaged membranes and set up fatty plaques. In fact, when you look even more carefully at the difference between small, dense LDL and large, buoyant LDL (the so-called pattern A type), the interesting difference is that large, buoyant LDL is much more enriched with fat than the smaller, dense LDL. My theory is that the larger amounts of fat in large, buoyant LDL protects the fat from excessive oxidation.

So we must be even more specific when we talk of fat. Not all fat is bad—there is good fat and bad fat. (In the 'Achieve optimum nutrition' chapter I will highlight the importance of good fat and how it protects us from all manner of diseases.) As with everything, it is vital to have balance in all aspects of our life, and what we eat is no exception. I must reinforce the fact that most of the evidence about the worth of reducing dietary fat is rather weak. There is no benefit from overall mortality and a rather weak benefit in regard to cardiovascular events.

The obsession with cholesterol lowering through rigid, boring diets really doesn't appear to be working; nor does it appear to be particularly relevent. In fact, when you look more carefully at fat intake, the biggest issue appears to be the intake of trans fatty acids. There is a close association between synthetic fats in the form of trans fatty acids, processed carbohydrates, both in the form of simple or complex sugars and the increasing use of food additives. These are the three major components of synthetic foods and all of them contribute to altering normal cellular metabolism. When we think of optimum health, we must consider the Cell Factor. Every time we ingest one of these synthetic foods, we are altering and deteriorating our cellular health. The first step in restoring cellular health through the Cell Factor is to minimise our exposure to synthetic foods that are damaging and destroying our membranes, the factory floor (known as the cytoplasm) and, of course, the control room—our nuclei.

LYON DIET HEART STUDY

This study was initially to run for five years and involved a group of 600 men from France who had survived a heart attack. Three hundred of them were advised to follow a prudent Western-style diet—a low-fat, high-carbohydrate diet. The other group were advised to follow a Mediterranean diet, which was enriched with alpha linolenic acid (the plant-based version of the Omega-3 fatty acids) essentially in the form of margarine that was high in canola oil. In short, the very simple diet suggested eating more whole-grain bread, more root and green vegetables, more fish, less beef, lamb and pork (replaced with poultry), fruit on a daily basis, and replacing butter and cream with the margarine high in alpha linolenic acid.

After two years, the trial was interrupted because of the amazing results: in those consuming the Mediterranean diet there was a 75 per cent reduction in all death and all cardiac events.

The trial was then continued for a further five years with around 400 participants, half of whom were on the Mediterranean diet and the other half on the low-fat diet, as before. Similar results were shown: a 65 per cent reduction in cardiac deaths, a 72 per cent in all cardiac events and a 56 per cent reduction in total mortality.

There is no single drug or surgical procedure that has these benefits. And these results were recorded despite the fact that the average cholesterol level at the end of the trial in both groups was around 6.2 millimoles per litre, with a slightly higher triglyceride value in the Mediterranean diet group of 1.9 as opposed to 1.75, and identical HDL levels of 1.3.

TRANS FATTY ACIDS

Trans fatty acids come from two major sources. Probably 10 per cent of the intake of trans fatty acids are found naturally in products from ruminant (cud-chewing) animals. Bacteria in the stomach of these animals, such as beef and dairy cattle, breaks down and in the process mixes hydrogen with some of the natural fats. The other source is from processed foods. These contribute about 90 per cent of the trans fatty acids in the average Western diet.

A large 10-year population study performed in Holland, known as the Zutphen Elderly Study, showed the more profound effect trans fatty acids had than saturated fat. It has been estimated that a 5 per cent increase in energy intake from saturated fat increases the risk for cardiac disease by about 17 per cent. When the Zutphen study pooled its data with three other studies, there was a 25 per cent decrease in risk when trans fatty acids were decreased. The largest study involved was the Nurses' Health Study. Around 80 000 nurses studied for over 15 years showed that the risk of having cardiac disease with a high trans fatty acid intake was more like 60 per cent. Some analyses even indicate that a 2 per cent increase in energy intake from trans fatty acids can increase the risk for cardiac disease by 93 per cent!

I, therefore, feel it is more important to put our emphasis on trans fatty acids than on the more natural saturated fats that we derive from meat products, such as red meat, chicken, pork and dairy products. I believe the central issue in the prevention of cardiovascular disease and, probably, cancer as far as our nutrition goes, is the synthetic poisons that are so prevalent in our foods today.

Trans fatty acids manifest their deleterious effects through the following five mechanisms:

1. By damaging the normal membrane of cells, therefore strongly affecting the cells' ability to take in appropriate nutrition. Membrane damage also affects electrolyte balance in the body, increasing irriability in that cell and in organs such as the heart, increasing the risk for sudden cardiac death.

2. By having a similar ability to raise LDL cholesterol as saturated fat.
3. Unlike saturated fat, however, trans fatty acids drop HDL cholesterol, further increasing the risk for cardiovascular disease.
4. Trans fatty acids also elevate lipoprotein(a) levels.
5. Trans fatty acids block the normal metabolism and distribution of Omega-3 fats, which are vital for good health.

Returning to the subject of optimum cell therapy, it is vital we maintain the health of all aspects of our cellular function. Once we introduce a diet loaded with trans fatty acids and processed carbohydrates, our first line of defence—the cell membrane—is attacked by the trans fatty acids. The trans fatty acids incorporate into the membrane. A diet high in trans fatty acids is usually low in the essential fatty acids (which I will discuss in the nutrition section). Trans fatty acids reduce the smooth, lubricated nature of the normal healthy membrane, and the membrane becomes much more rigid and also prevents the normal flow of surface proteins, which act as receptors. As I have already mentioned, it is vital for these processes to be functioning normally.

A recent study from Washington showed that high levels of trans fatty acids in the bloodstream were associated with a threefold increase in risk of sudden cardiac death. The reason for this is that if your membranes are clogged with trans fatty acids, the normal messages to the heart are corrupted and the heart becomes very irritable, especially as the fat builds up in the system. Thus, if you have a heart attack, you are more likely to die suddenly if the levels of trans fatty acids are high in your bloodstream. The trans fatty acids also block the ability of good fats to get into the membrane. Basically, these horrible trans fatty acids clog up the membrane so much that nutrients find it very difficult to reach all aspects of the cell, including the nucleus, and cellular function goes out the window.

It is excessive consumption of these trans fatty acids that contributes significantly to us feeling constantly tired, having a poor immune system and the ongoing rampage to our bodies from cardiac disease and cancer. It's no wonder many of us feel quite unhealthy, develop recurring infections, lack energy and eventually develop chronic diseases as we age. But the story does not stop there. If you do not have a normally functioning membrane and the nutrients are not getting into the cells, your energy supplies are, therefore, depleted. What then happens is you crave carbohydrates because your cells are perceiving that they are not getting enough glucose. When you have a diet that is high in carbohydrates, especially processed carbohydrates, these excess chemicals rapidly turn to triglycerides and are stored in our body as fat. We have been mistaken for too long that it is fat that becomes fat. There is, of course, an element of truth in this, but nowhere near to the extent that carbohydrates, if they are not burned immediately as they enter the body, are altered to contribute to that enormous envelope of fat you may be seeing increasing around your abdomen.

The consequences of excessive carbohydrates are very concerning: marked abdominal obesity, an epidemic of diabetes, predisposition to high blood pressure, and a moderate elevation in cholesterol, high triglycerides and a low HDL cholesterol. One of my good friends has recently been diagnosed as diabetic. He is in his late forties, is significantly obese and is hypertensive. His cholesterol level is only 5 millimoles per litre and he is quite proud of this. He was unaware (until I told him) that his triglycerides, which are 3, and his HDL, which is 1, pose an enormous risk for his insulin resistance syndrome and his excessive carbohydrate consumption—rampant cardiovascular disease. Once we rid our bodies of trans fatty acids and improve our intake of essential fatty acids, our carbohydrate addiction soon disappears. We find we no longer have this enormous craving for carbohydrates because our cells are working under optimum conditions rather than sluggishly groaning along as they have been doing for many years.

In short, the human body, and in particular our cells, was not designed to tolerate synthetic chemicals. Our modern lifestyle, which is so chemcially based, is really the main cause for the major diseases common in our society. If we examine all the common afflictions of modern society we see that, at each level in our body, these diseases are closely related to exposure to trans fatty acids, processed carbohydrates and other chemicals added to the food.

The outer covering of the body, affectionately known as the skin, is the first line of exposure to these synthetic chemicals. Chronic skin disorders are rampant in our society and, in many cases, are due to some type of reaction to some type of chemical. One interesting example is the common affliction of teenagers. Many teenagers are fast-food, soft-drink junkies and often exist on diets that make their more health-conscious parents cringe. These diets are, of course, loaded with trans fatty acids, processed carbohydrates and other food additives. In my opinion, this is the major reason for them developing quite significant acne. It is often the acne rather than the long-term health consequences that makes a teenager change their diet.

The next part of our body exposed to all of these dangerous chemicals is, of course, our lungs. As we don't tend to breathe in trans fatty acids, processed carbohydrates or food additives, it is probably more relevant to talk about the damaging effects of inhaled pollutants, such as cigarette smoke and general pollution. The lungs that must receive all of our blood supply because it is through the lungs that the blood picks up oxygen. The cells lining the air sacks (known as the alveoli) are prone to problems from inhaled pollutants as well as from trans fatty acids, processed carbohydrates and additives, as are all the other cells in the body. All these compound the problems.

The next area significantly affected by all of these poisons is, of course, our gastrointestinal tract. From our mouth to our anus we have cells that are involved in the digestion, absorption and the excretion of food and fluid. These cells function like any other cells in the body—they require a constant and healthy supply of nutrients. They are just as prone to membrane damage, cytoplasm damage and nuclear damage as any other cell in the body and need a constant, ongoing supply of essential fatty acids, natural fats and other nutrients to perform their expected tasks.

Modern society is plagued with dyspepsia, peptic ulceration and irritable colon. Many doctors put this all down to stress. I am not denying there is a strong stress component, but I also believe there is a strong nutritional component. The altered membrane function along the lining of the gastrointestinal tract damages local immunity and allows bacteria, such as Helicobacter (felt to be the main cause of peptic ulceration and possibly gastric and oesophageal cancer), to set up an infective focus and cause its mischief. It is highly likely that reducing our exposure to these chronic nutritional poisons will stop Helicobacter from putting its foot in the door of the gastrointestinal tract and setting up camp for what for Helicobacter would be a long and happy association. But for the person so infected, it reminds me of what Oscar Wilde once said about house guests: 'House guests are like fish, they go off after two or three days.' And I would suggest that anybody who invites Helicobacter into their body through excessive doses of these chronic nutritional poisons will feel the same after being plagued by chronic indigestion, peptic ulceration, and the possibility of all sorts of nasty cancers.

At present, the way we are dealing with Helicobacter is to give people a course of triple antibiotic therapy for a week or so, donging the bug on the head. This certainly may rid the body of Helicobacter temporarily, and at times permanently, but doesn't really solve the problem of what allowed Helicobacter to be there in the first place.

There is a growing body of gastroenterologists who also believe that irritable colon syndrome has an inflammatory basis. This may or may not be the case but I certainly believe that better nutrition and better stress management will help relieve and, in some cases, completely abolish the symptoms of bowel problems. Once these chronic nutritional poisons penetrate the gastrointestinal tract into our bloodstream they are delivered to every cell in the body.

Thus, concentrating on my field of cardiovascular disease, there are numerous studies showing a very close and strong relationship between trans fatty acid intake and the intake of processed carbohydrates as a major factor in the generation of cardiovascular disease.

WHY FOOD PRODUCERS USE TRANS FATTY ACIDS

One of the great con jobs of the food industry is products that claim to be cholesterol-free, low in saturated fat and free of animal fats. What these manufacturers fail to tell you is that they are using mono-unsaturated fats (such as olive oil or polyunsaturated fats, which are usually liquid at room temperature. A process, known as chemical hydrogenation of these unsaturated oils, changes them into the trans fatty acid configuration. This makes them solid and easy to use extensively in different types of processed and fast foods. While ensuring the foods are more solid, they also ensure a greater resistance to oxidation and rancidity, providing much longer shelf lives. Just imagine, if they are added to foods to keep them on the shelf for longer, what happens to these chemicals once they get into your body?

Trans fatty acids in restaurant foods

Fried foods	Calories	Total fat (g)	Trans fat (g)
Onion rings (8 rings—170 grams)	650	47	7
Burger King french fries (king-size—170 grams)	540	24	7
McDonald's chicken nuggets (9 pieces)	510	29	3
McDonald's french fries (large—142 grams)	470	19	4
Fried mozzarella sticks (4 sticks—113 grams)	370	23	3
Fried fish (170 grams)	350	16	3
Miscellaneous foods			
Prime rib, untrimmed (170 grams precooked weight)	480	35	3
Hamburger (142 grams)	470	26	2
Chicken pot pie (198 grams)	370	20	3
KFC biscuit (57 grams)	210	12	4
Pastries and desserts			
Cinnabon cinnabun (226 grams)	670	34	6
Apple pie (99 grams)	236	12	3

The problem with trans fatty acids first came to light when the most common form of trans fatty acids, known as elaidic acid (the 'trans' form of the most common mono-unsaturated fat, oleic acid), was found to increase LDL cholesterol and reduce HDL cholesterol. This particular substance also increased lipoprotein(a). The Nurses' Health Study showed clearly how the consumption of foods high in elaidic acid (usually certain types of margarine) increased the risk of heart disease by 50 per cent. Elaidic acid occurs when either fish oils or vegetable oils are hydrogenated to form the older style of margarines and shortenings used to thicken processed and takeaway foods.

In Europe, fish oils are commonly used in processed foods but not so in Australia. Hydrogenated fish oils in Europe and the hydrogenated vegetable oils in Australia are used as a shortening for all forms of pastries, biscuits, hamburger rolls and other different types of processed foods. Elaidic acid is a cheap form of processed fat with a much longer shelf life than natural fats.

In different parts of India and Pakistan they use an oil known as Vanaspathi, which is high in trans fatty acids. Interestingly, in the areas where it is used, there are corresponding high levels of coronary heart disease.

Types of foods containing trans fatty acids

Until recently, 50 per cent of the fat found in margarine was in the trans fatty acid form. With the newer margarines, such as the olive oil–canola oil combinations or the new plant sterol-based cholesterol-lowering margarines, the trans fatty acids are now less than 1 per cent.

The other sources of trans fatty acids are also sources of significant processed carbohydrates—crackers and cookies, croissants, potato chips and french fries, cakes and pancake mixes along with waffles and doughnuts are all loaded with trans fatty acids. Unfortunately, around 3 to 5 grams of trans fatty acids can be found in a single serving of many processed and fast-food products. The average intake in Western society of trans fatty acids ranges somewhere between 6 and 15 grams per person per day.

If your trans fatty acid intake is around 9 grams a day, this equates to around 4 per cent of total energy in trans fatty acids. It is fairly obvious that the younger population is consuming much more than this.

Food products are now often labelled with the amount of total fat, saturated fat, mono-unsaturated fat and polyunsaturated fats. Some food manufacturers are honest enough to put the content of trans fatty acids on the side of the packet, but it is usually the foods that are loaded with trans fatty acids whose packaging conveniently omits this vital information. The next time you decide to munch on whatever your favourite nibbly is, be very mindful of the fact that probably at least 50 per cent of the total fat in that product is in the form of trans fatty acids. This is the problem and there is a solution: avoid them!

PROCESSED CARBOHYDRATES

Walk into almost any book store and you will see a multitude of diet books. Those written by members of the conservative medical or nutrition profession will laud the benefits of a low-fat, high-carbohydrate diet. Some more adventurous people will discuss a *good*-fat, high-carbohydrate diet. The more controversial authors, such as Dr Robert Atkins and the numerous spin-offs, talk about the benefits of a high-protein, low-carbohydrate diet. While we should not be completely depriving ourselves of carbohydrates, it is much more sensible to have a balanced diet.

We need at least 50 to 100 grams of carbohydrate per day to ensure normal fat metabolism. Most of our daily carbohydrate intake should come from fruit and vegetables. Scientific research into communities and countries consuming significant amounts of fruit and vegetables have shown a much lower risk of heart disease and cancer. The global benefits of fruit and vegetables are enormous and I would be very wary of any diet that does not promote their use. Fruits and vegetables have mainly carbohydrates as their main macronutrient, except for occasional products such as the wonderful avocado, which is almost all fat with little carbohydrate.

We are having far too much in the way of processed carbohydrates in our diet, and I would like to divide these into simple carbohydrates and complex carbohydrates.

Simple carbohydrates

The simple carbohydrates are glucose, fructose and galactose. Almost all of the simple and complex carbohydrates are eventually broken down to glucose in the body.

One teaspoonful of sugar is the equivalent of 5 grams of carbohydrate. Table sugar is basically sucrose, which is half glucose and half natural fructose. It is my opinion, that simple sugar is not as bad for you as the simple carbohydrate derived from high-fructose corn syrups, which are a cheap source of sweetener made through treating corn starch with acid and enzymes. In the United States especially, this is the major source of sweetening in desserts, lollies, jam, jelly and soft drinks. Most breakfast cereals are also sweetened with this high-fructose corn syrup. Fructose is closely related to glucose and is found in either fruit, honey, or this rather disturbing high-fructose corn syrup.

There are two areas that need further discussion. First, the fructose in fruit is in a lower dose than the excessive amount in high-fructose corn syrup. Therefore, we are not flooding our bodies with fructose when we eat fruit and we are also benefiting from all of the other wonderful phyto-chemicals present in fruit, along with the excellent fibre. The high-fructose corn syrup comes in much higher concentrations and has little other nutrient value, apart from the obvious sweetness.

The more disturbing area is that fructose is present in two forms. It comes as either the natural furanose five-ring structure, or the more stable synthetic pyranose six-ring structure. It may well be that the six-ring structure, being more stable, is more difficult for the body to break down and may even block some of the normal glucose metabolic pathways. Further research needs to be done on this concept.

The average American diet over the past 30 years has seen a significant drop in saturated fat and cholesterol. Interestingly, however, with this reduction in saturated fat there has been a marked increase in dietary fructose, especially from the high-fructose corn syrup, as possibly the major sweetener in the average American diet. High-fructose corn syrup is not a major factor in Australian food products, the most common sweeteners being sugar or fruit concentrates. Fructose has been shown to increase LDL cholesterol: increasing dietary fructose from 3 to 20 per cent of calories increases total cholesterol 9 per cent and LDL cholesterol 11 per cent. Simply put, a 2 per cent increase in dietary fructose raises LDL cholesterol by greater than 1 per cent. Dietary fructose has also been shown to promote atherosclerosis more than any other carbohydrate. One study found that the haemoglobin, A1-C, which is an indication of glucose control, was damaged seven times faster with fructose than with glucose.

One of the interesting explanations for fructose's more concerning effects than glucose is that when fructose enters the liver, it bypasses a particular enzyme, thus it is more readily converted to fat than glucose. It is now estimated that around 10 per cent of the energy consumption in food in the United States is in fructose-based sweeteners.

A recent study of a particular type of hamster with a very similar metabolism to humans showed that a high-fructose diet caused insulin resistance and a high triglyceride level in the hampsters. Therefore it was fructose causing this predisposition to diabetes, and not simple sugar. In another study of two-dozen healthy human volunteers, those consuming a diet of 17 per cent fructose had a marked increase in their triglyceride levels compared with a normal glucose diet.

It, therefore, may be these cheap forms of sweetening rather than glucose itself that is causing this rampant increase in insulin resistance. Isn't it interesting how many of the foods using this highly processed carbohydrate are the same foods containing trans fatty acids? Do you see a trend here?

HIGH VERSUS LOW GLYCAEMIC INDEX FOODS

It may shock you to know that a baked potato is among the highest glycaemic index foods. The entire concept of high versus low glycaemic index foods is based around how quickly it takes blood sugar to respond to carbohydrates. Interestingly, some of the high glycaemic index foods include short-grain rice, baked potato, honey, bagels, white bread, high-energy sports drinks and different types of wafers.

Glycemic index (GI) of common foods

Reference food (glucose) = 100
Low GI foods—below 55
Intermediate GI foods—between
55 and 70
High GI foods—more than 70

Sugars	
Honey	73
Sucrose	65
Fructose	23
Lactose	46

Pastas/grains	
Brown rice	55
White, long-grain	56
White, short-grain	72
Spaghetti	41

Breads and muffins	
Bagel	72
Whole-wheat bread	69
White bread	70
Croissant	67

Vegetables	
Carrots, boiled	49
Sweet corn	55
Potato, baked	85
New (red) potato, boiled	62

Fruits	
Apple	38
Banana	55
Grapefruit	25
Orange	44

Dairy foods	
Milk, whole	27
Milk, skim	32
Yogurt, low-fat	33
Ice cream	61

Beverages	
Apple juice	40
Orange juice	46
Gatarade	78
Coca-Cola	63

Legumes	
Baked beans	48
Kidney beans	27
Lentils	30
Navy beans	38

Snack foods	
Potato chips	54
Vanilla wafers	77
Chocolate	49
Jelly beans	80

Adapted from J. Brand-Miller, T. Wolever, S. Calagiuri & K. Foster-Powell, *The Glucose Revolution—The Authoritative Guide to the Glycemic Index*, New York: Marlowe & Company, 1999.

I believe this is somewhat simplistic as it gives people the impression that high glycaemic index carbohydrates cause much more concern than the low glycaemic carbohydrates. But fructose has a very low glycaemic index of only 23, as opposed to 73 for honey and 65 for simple sugar. If we purely rely on the glycaemic index of these foods, then fructose should not be causing us much in the way of bother whatsoever. Also, whole milk, for example, has a lower glycaemic index than skim milk. A banana, which is high in potassium and fibre, has a glycaemic index of 55—rather close to that of ice cream (61) and Coca-Cola (63). I, therefore, feel that foods with attached glycaemic indices add more confusion than help us decide what we should be consuming. To rely purely on a blood glucose response to a particular food does not consider the fact that if the foods are absorbed, they will still eventually contribute to the glucose load in the body and, therefore, promote the production of insulin.

The third major simple carbohydrate is galactose, which is basically found in milk. Galactose is usually not found alone, it combines with glucose to form lactose. Many members of the community, especially the Asian community, are lactose-intolerant because they lack an enzyme known as lactase, which breaks down the lactose to allow absorption. This lactose intolerance can lead to marked intestinal gas, bloating, cramping and discomfort.

Simple sugars of any variety tend to raise the blood sugar level quite rapidly. One of the issues these days is the fluid intake of children and teenagers.

When I was a child, the government used to supply bottles of milk for us to have for morning tea. Often, we would drink the milk after it had been left in the sun for half an hour or so. It was so warm that afterwards we'd usually go and find a convenient place to throw up.

On a more serious note, the fact that milk was our major fluid intake meant we were getting a strong source of calcium for our growing bones. These days, children have either soft drinks or fruit juices, both of which are loaded with processed sugars and certainly contain no calcium. Even more concerning is the cola-based drinks containing phosphoric acid which tends to leech calcium out of the bones. Because of this rather disturbing trend, we are seeing increasing numbers of people in their late thirties and early forties with osteoporosis. I am, of course, not blaming the simple carbohydrates for this, but it is the sweetness that attracts the person to the drink and, of course, the companies that produce soft drinks and fruit juices are not going to stress the lack of calcium or the calcium-leeching effects of some of these drinks.

It is my feeling that soft drinks are better seen as a weekly treat rather than a daily method of encouraging fluid intake. If fruit juices are to be taken at all, I would suggest they are diluted in water.

ARTIFICIAL SWEETENERS

Many people, especially diabetics, have taken to using alternative sweeteners. Institutions, such as the World Health Organization and many diabetic associations are strong supporters of these alternative sweeteners. The most common types of sweeteners used these days are saccharin and aspartame. Saccharin, at one stage, was thought to cause cancer in laboratory animals, but this has never been proven in a large human population and it continues to be used as a sweetener. Aspartame is the usual sweetener for diet drinks and is a combination of phenylalanine and aspartic acid, along with methanol. (This actually sounds like a rather potent combination to me.) Although there have been some reported reactions to aspartame, it is felt that the numbers are relatively low and there has been no good evidence to suggest a link between cancer and this particular artificial sweetener. Sufferers of the extremely rare condition known as phenylketonuria should certainly not take any foodstuff that has had aspartame added.

I cannot give an opinion either way as to whether I believe sweeteners are safe. My attitude to this entire discussion is if it has been manufactured rather than harvested from nature, there is still some concern as to its long-term effects. It may be completely harmless, but I do not believe that anyone can honestly say yes or no.

Complex carbohydrates

We can divide complex carbohydrates into two main groups:

1. digestible (which includes starch and glycogen)
2. indigestible (which are the dietary fibres).

Complex carbohydrates in the digestible form come from plants as either amylose or amylopectin. Amylopectin raises blood sugar much more rapidly than amylose because it is branched, therefore the body can break it down much more easily. In most typical complex carbohydrates, amylose to amylopectin is in a ratio of about 1:4.

The common sources of these complex carbohydrates are foods such as cereal, pasta, rice, bread and potatoes. We have been told for far too long that our diet should contain significant amounts of these five sources of complex carbohydrates but often, after a few sandwiches of white bread, the blood sugar can rise just as much as having a bowl of ice cream. I am not suggesting we eliminate these from our diet, but I believe we do not need more than two or three pieces of bread per day, and when we have rice or pasta, we should limit the amount that we ingest.

Before you purchase a cereal, read the carbohydrate content on the packet. If there is more than 15 grams per serve, I would avoid it. Of course, if you are going to eat bread, I would strongly suggest wholegrain bread or the new soy-and-linseed variety—try to avoid too much in the way of white bread, bread rolls and other highly processed forms of bread.

There are numerous types of dietary fibre that add bulk to the faeces and decrease intestinal transit times. The major sources of fibre in the diet are fruits, vegetables, legumes (in the form of beans, lentils or peas, nuts and seeds, and wholegrains and cereals). Beans are not only an excellent source of fibre—and have been the brunt of many jokes in famous film scenes—but also have wonderful proteins that are very beneficial in maintaining good health. One apple contains around 4 grams of fibre; half a cup of some form of legumes is anywhere between 5 and 7 grams of fibre. The fibre content of different types of breads is variable but information can usually be obtained from the side of the container.

One of the problems with diets along the high-protein, low-carbohydrate line is the obvious loss of dietary fibre from a reduction in fruit, vegetables and legumes. Many people starting on one of these diets have developed acute haemorrhoids and severe constipation. A diet high in dietary fibre leads to large, soft stools as different forms of plant fibre attract water. Two large studies, one in men and one in women, showed ingesting somewhere between 20 and 35 grams of fibre per day also reduced the risk of coronary heart disease in the 30 to 40 per cent range.

By consuming three to five servings of vegetables per day, along with two or three pieces of fruit, some nuts, two to three slices of wholegrain (or soy-and-linseed) bread, with or without legumes, it is not difficult to reach somewhere between 20 and 35 grams of fibre per day.

ACRYLAMIDE AND CANCER

At some stage in their nutritional career, most foods have been claimed to cause cancer. Those of us who enjoy our meat extremely well done are well aware of the potential cancer effect from the nitrosamines. Many chemically produced foods, such as commercial peanut butters and margarines, have also been implicated in some animal studies as a potential cause for cancer. Just recently a study at Stockholm University in Sweden showed high concentrations of acrylamide were produced when carbohydrate-rich foods, such as rice, potatoes and cereals, are fried or baked. The headlines came out: 'Carbohydrates Cause Cancer'.

Acrylamide is released as a result of baking or frying. It seems now for many years we have been consuming acrylamide in biscuits, bread and french fries. Interestingly, the amounts of acrylamide range from 350 to 3500 parts per billion in different varieties of chips. In the chips that are over-cooked, however, this rises to 12 000 parts per billion. Acrylamide is even found in foods cooked at high temperatures, such as rye biscuits. On the other hand, no levels of acrylamide were found in raw or boiled foods.

Acrylamide has been found to cause gene mutations leading to specific cancers in laboratory animals, such as breast cancer, uterine cancer, and tumour in the adrenal glands and the scrotum. These tumours, however, occur at much higher concentrations of acrylamide than seen in the fried or baked foods. This very much gets back to the age-old question, what is a safe level of poison? and stresses the fact that the more natural the food, the less the risk. The body was certainly not designed to take in all these synthetic and synthetically changed foods.

ADDITIVES

Major food companies make billions of dollars each year from processed packaged food. Food that can sit on the shelf for a few months (or in many cases, even longer) allows mass production and is obviously more convenient for all of us living in this fast-paced world. One of the major problems with this approach is the amount of extra chemicals needed to increase the nutrient content or shelf life and also to make the food more palatable. Some of these additives are clearly harmful to some people (such as the sulphites), and other additives can accidentally make it into foods.

Recently in Australia, there has been significant publicity given to the heavy contamination of our soil transferring into many foodstuffs by a whole host of toxic poisons. How many of these occurrences occur all over the world and go completely unnoticed and unpublicised?

If you believe or listen to the conspiracy theories, our domestic animals are dripping with pesticides, bacteria, antibiotics, hormones and numerous other chemicals that can cause many of the major diseases that lead to our downfall. If, however, you consider these people abject loonies and you are very comfortable believing the government and manufacturers, along with the numerous food and drug administrations throughout the world, you will ingest your processed, packaged foods or your meat and dairy with the same loving trust a baby has for its mother's breast. Many cancer researchers would suggest that there are many more natural toxins than there are synthetic poisons in food. To use the old argument, snakebite is entirely natural but can kill you within minutes.

One of the major reasons for food additives is to allow food to sit on the shelf for months at a time. The additives limit food spoilage through reducing the growth of different bacteria and fungi, and they also preserve an acceptable colour and flavour. Much of this is accomplished by different types of preservatives in the form of vitamins and sulphites.

These are intentional food additives but unfortunately there are also incidental food additives as well.

Most of the accepted food additives have been tested on either rats or mice but not all diseases occurring or not occurring in these types of laboratory animals will occur in human beings. Most of us will consume on a daily basis multiple different types of food that cannot really be seen as natural. Because we are exposed to thousands and thousands of micro doses of different chemicals over a prolonged period of time, no-one can really be sure which agent is related to which disease process—if at all. One of the problems with the diseases, such as heart diesease and cancer, is the environment–organism interaction. In the case of some chemical additive in food, this may be ingested for many years before it causes a problem, and because there are so many different additives and so many different foods, we may have absolutely no idea and in fact, never find out that this particular additive caused a problem. This is regardless of how much testing has been performed by the food industry and regardless of who does the testing.

In many ways we have to adopt the philosophy that life is a risk. We take a risk every time we venture out of our house into some form of private or public transport. In most cases we will survive this transport risk but we hear almost on a daily basis of someone being killed in a car accident, a train crash or multiple deaths from a large commercial airliner crashing somewhere in some part of the world.

Cardiovascular disease

Cardiovascular disease is the biggest killer in our society, accounting for around 45 per cent of deaths. The majority of these deaths are due to atherosclerosis in either the coronary arteries or the cerebral arteries. These fatty plaques rupture to cause either heart attack or stroke—depending on the site of the atherosclerosis. One in four people will die of a heart attack. Unfortunately, 30 per cent of heart attack deaths are sudden and without warning.

Although we have made great advances in the treatment of cardiovascular disease, we are still not winning the fight. Ongoing research into all areas of medicine is vital, but I believe we have many answers already that can minimise our future risk for all manner of diseases.

The following case studies demonstrate the broad nature of cardiovascular disease.

Case study: Dr James Wright—My friend and colleague Dr James Wright is a legend in Australian medicine. In many ways, he single-handedly created a human side to the medical profession through his appearances in the media. Behind the public face is a man who works tirelessly for the community. Despite being in his seventies, he has more energy than most people in their forties. You may be surprised to hear that Dr Wright still studies and reviews medical journals for at least one hour a day and has a very intricate system to retrieve his enormous knowledge base. This system was created long before computers were ever thought of.

Dr Wright has long been a health fanatic, treating his body with the same care that he approaches all of his numerous projects. In 1999, he was one of the first to make an appointment for a screen of his coronary arteries. This revolutionary new test uses a very high-speed CT scan of the coronary arteries in between heart-beats, when the heart is moving least. Basically, the test assesses for coronary artery calcium, which has been shown in numerous scientific studies to be an accurate marker for the degree of fat in the arteries. Simply put, the more calcium, the more fat; and therefore the more risk of some sort of cardiac event, such as severe angina, heart attack or, worse, sudden cardiac death.

When Dr Wright went through the CT scanner his score was 48. For a man of 72 this was an excellent score but his cholesterol was around 6 millimoles per litre. Being an absolute perfectionist, Dr Wright wasn't happy that he'd scored any calcium at all, and certainly wasn't happy with his cholesterol level.

He then tightened his lifestyle even further (and I'm not particularly sure how he did that!), consumed more antioxidant dose vitamins, and began taking Atorvastatin (a very strong cholesterol lowering agent). He returned two years later for a repeat CT scan to determine his progress. Comparable images were obtained showing the score of 48 had shrunk down to a small dot of 6 in the same place. His arteries looked smoother and there was certainly no evidence of any new plaques developing.

It is quite remarkable that definite reversal of coronary artery disease was demonstrated in a man in his early seventies. But this is proof-positive that you can achieve reversal of heart disease if you really want to.

Case study: John—John was 45 years old and a very busy executive who spent more time on his business than on his health and his family life. Because of this he was separated from his wife. Despite the obvious traumas this caused his family, he continued to work hard. He was only slightly overweight with a cholesterol of 5.8 millimoles per litre, a HDL (good cholesterol) of 1.2, a triglyceride level of 2.4 and his blood sugar was 6. He had stopped smoking at the age of 38 and his blood pressure was slightly elevated at 135/90.

John's father had died of a heart attack at the age of 53 and John's mother was diabetic.

He'd heard about CT scanning of the coronary arteries and thought, with his history and obvious risk factors, it wouldn't be a bad idea for him to have one. However, every time he made an appointment (which was on three occasions), an important business meeting came up and he had to cancel. Eventually, he could keep an appointment, and his results showed a score of 450, which placed him at a very high risk for a man of his age. Although John was tired, he had no definite symptoms. The doctor strongly suggested further testing with stress-echocardiography, but John had to rush off to yet another important business meeting.

Over the weekend John died suddenly. It may be called 'sudden', but what is sudden about a man who continually cancels appointments despite having an obvious need to be assessed? Is there really any meeting that is more important than one that is beneficial to your health—in John's case, life-savingly so?

Case study: Sri Chatterjee—Sri Chatterjee is a 62-year-old Fijian-Indian lady who was referred to me with left-sided chest tightness that occurred inconsistently with exercise. On further questioning, however, I discovered that it was unusual for Sri to do any exercise at all. Simple housework was enough to give her this left-sided discomfort and it also did not take much for her to become extremely short of breath.

Sri had been diagnosed as diabetic 10 years ago. Her blood pressure was constantly a problem, usually sitting at 160/100. Her endocrinologist informed her that the cholesterol was quite good but on further examination, while her total cholesterol was 5, her triglycerides were 3.6 and her HDL was 1. I would consider this a very concerning lipid (or fat) profile. Fortunately, she had never smoked but two of her brothers had had bypass surgery and her father had died of a heart attack when in his fifties. Most of her relatives were non-insulin dependent diabetics.

Sri had tried numerous low-fat diets and despite her greatest efforts, had progressively gained weight over the past 15 years since menopause. She had quite significant arthritis in her right knee, which made exercise very difficult, so I performed a test known as a dobutamine stress echocardiogram. After the early stages of intravenous dobutamine (a drug that simulates exercise, making the heart work harder and faster) she developed her left-sided chest pain and became very short of breath. At the same time, a large part of her heart stopped working on the echocardiogram (ultrasound of the heart) despite the fact that the electrocardiogram (indication of the electrical activity of the heart) did not show any abnormalities.

I organised for a semi-urgent angiogram to be performed, which showed high-grade blockages in most of her major coronary arteries. Sri then went on to have successful coronary artery bypass grafting but that was only the start of her road to recovery. Unfortunately, in Western society, we consider bypass as a curative procedure; in fact, it is a temporary procedure until we can get our life in order. The way to treat blockages in the arteries is to either unblock them with stents or balloons, or to bypass them with surgery. This however, does not treat the underlying process, which is atherosclerosis. Atherosclerosis needs a very intensive reversal program, otherwise the process will recur in the grafted vessels.

So what risk factors should alert you to this higher possibility of cardiovascular disease? I would like to divide these into 'traditional' risk factors and 'newer' risk factors.

Traditional factors include:

- cholesterol and related abnormalities
- hypertension
- cigarette smoking
- diabetes
- family history.

The newer risk factors include:

- lipoprotein(a)
- homocysteine
- highly sensitive C-reactive protein (hs-CRP)
- inflammatory states (in particular, infections)
- thrombotic (pro-clotting) states.

CHOLESTEROL AND RELATED ABNORMALITIES

If you asked the man on the street what the most common cause of heart disease is, he would probably answer, 'Cholesterol'. When people think of cholesterol they think of some sort of dreadful disease. They say, 'I've got cholesterol', as if it were something like leprosy. Possibly, people think you 'catch' cholesterol from hanging around outside takeaway-food outlets.

Cholesterol is a vital nutrient essential for life. It is the most common form of sterol, the chemicals that are the basis of many natural components throughout the body. For example, all of the steroid hormones, such as cortisone and aldosterone, and the reproductive hormones, oestrogen, progesterone and testosterone, are formed from cholesterol. If your adrenal glands were removed and you were not given supplemental hormones, you would be dead within 24 hours.

Cholesterol is also a vital and normal part of every cell membrane in the body. It takes part in many of the normal cellular reactions and is thus essential to our wellbeing. So why all the concern regarding cholesterol? you may well ask.

Firstly, we probably don't require more than around 3 millimoles of cholesterol per litre of blood for normal existence. In rural China the average cholesterol level sits somewhere between 2 and 3 millimoles per litre throughout life, and these people certainly do not develop significant atherosclerotic disease (a build-up of plaque in the arteries). Basically, they use all their cholesterol for normal cellular metabolism. The human body was designed for this type of nourishment. When you are exposed to a lifelong, Western diet, however, it is extremely rare to have a cholesterol reading below this range.

I personally analyse thousands of cholesterol results per year and only very occasionally would see a level below 3, unless people are taking cholesterol-lowering pills. Once the cholesterol level starts to rise above 3, then the risk for significant atherosclerosis occurs. If you examine the arteries of people dying below the age of 30 in Western society for non-cardiac reasons, such as accidents, suicide or cancer, around 80 per cent already have substantial fat build-up in their arteries due to the Western diet.

Secondly, any fat in your arteries creates the potential for fatty plaque to rupture and cause a heart attack. Usually and most consistently, the more fat, the more risk you have; but during my long career I've still seen quite a number of patients with relatively normal arteries who have had quite substantial heart attacks. I have also seen a number of people below the age of 30 who have had heart attacks. So the big question is: what role does cholesterol play? My view is, although cholesterol is important, we have in many ways overemphasised its importance as a factor in heart disease.

When cholesterol first emerged as a major risk back in the 1960s and '70s, it was felt this was only of concern for people who had cholesterols well above 7 millimoles per litre. There is no doubt that people with cholesterols in this range are at a very high risk for some type of cardiac event. Usually people with cholesterols of this magnitude, as an isolated finding, have a condition known as familial hypercholesterolaemia, which is a strongly inherited cholesterol problem.

Even in our educated society I see many people with familial hypercholesterolaemia who lament the fact they have been on every diet and not one budged their cholesterol in any way, shape or form. I have seen people go to the extremes of following the Pritikin Diet, which shifted their cholesterol maybe from 8 down to 6 for a month or two, but a few months later the level drifted back to 8.

From the outset it is important to realise that only 25 per cent of the cholesterol in the body is related to food. The other 75 per cent is produced by the liver. If you have a strong genetic cholesterol-producing gene, no matter what goes in your mouth, you will not be able to control your cholesterol without some form of medication. This does not give you licence to eat whatever you like because if you do have this gene and you eat the type of diet I suggest you avoid, your cholesterol will go through the roof.

Case study: Malcolm Patterson—Malcolm Patterson was 26 years old. His cholesterol was 10 millimoles per litre, his HDL was 1 millimole per litre, and his triglycerides were normal at 0.7 millimoles per litre. His father died at age 32 of a heart attack. Malcolm worked in the financial industry, was highly intelligent and driven, and smoked from the age of 17. He enjoyed Friday evening drinks with the boys and weekend rugby during winter and cricket during summer.

He was a keen skier and over the Christmas break travelled to Whistler in Canada with a few of his friends. While skiing down one of the slopes he fell. When his mates realised he was not down with them they looked up to see many people gathering around his body—a few were attempting CPR, to no avail. Malcolm was dead at 26.

Malcolm suffered familial hypercholesterolaemia, and the combination of very bad genetics and a rather hectic lifestyle brought about a tragic premature demise. There is no doubt that with earlier detection of his problems and better management, Malcolm's life could have been saved. He is now yet another unfortunate cardiac statistic.

Around one in 500 people carry the gene for familial hypercholesterolaemia. With the advent of better cholesterol-lowering therapy, the manifestations of this gene can be controlled. This gene, however, is just one of the many reasons you should have an early medical check-up if you have a strong family history of premature heart disease. If you are, say, 20 and your father died in his thirties or forties from a heart attack, I would recommend you have a full cholesterol profile, along with an assessment of endothelial function with arterial tonometry (discussed later) to determine the health of your arteries and whether treatment is necessary.

In almost all cases such as these, it will be vital to follow very strict lifestyle principles, along with taking a cholesterol-lowering agent. As these drugs are very powerful metabolic agents, however, I suggest women in reproductive years, even with this family history, do not take the medications for three months prior to conceiving, for the entire pregnancy, and probably while you are breastfeeding. It is important to add that familial hypercholesterolaemia probably accounts for only less than 5 per cent of heart disease.

THE FRAMINGHAM STUDY

Just outside Boston in the US state of Massachusetts is a city known as Framingham. Around 50 years ago the Framingham Study commenced—every member of the community was tested for all kinds of common diseases and ailments and their medical conditions have been followed since then. Framingham has been a landmark study, especially for cardiovascular disease. What shocked the medical world following the initial enthusiasm regarding cholesterol in the '70s was the rather disconcerting fact that the average cholesterol level of heart-attack sufferers in Framingham was around 6.2 millimoles per litre—it was thought that cholesterols above 7 were the worry.

Further work from Framingham and other studies has shown that cholesterol abnormalities of some description really only explain around 35 per cent of coronary heart disease attack rates. It is far too simplistic to blame one factor on a condition that requires a multitude of stimuli to generate disease in the arteries. There was no doubt, however, that the combination of lifelong non-smoking, serum cholesterol levels below 5.17 and blood pressure readings below 120/80, offered striking benefits. If these three factors were present, the risk for coronary heart disease was extremely low. People in this category had life expectancy of 10 years longer than those considered to be of elevated risk.

In most of these studies, however, the number of people who were in this category was fewer than 10 per cent. Therefore, 90 per cent of the population is at varying risk for heart disease, depending on the numbers of risk factors present. If you are less than 40 years of age, a non-smoker with low cholesterol and blood pressure, your long-term risk for a cardiac event is 92 per cent less than those at high risk. If you are older than 40 with the same low-risk factors, you have around a 75 per cent reduction in risk.

Before delving further into the cholesterol story, I believe it is important to put the entire atherosclerosis subject into perspective. From the moment of conception we are exposed to a combination of genetic and environmental factors. If, for example, your mother or father had a genetic form of high cholesterol, your blood vessels could have already been primed with too much fat—even before you got your first peak at the sunshine. Some babies who died in utero were found to have a build-up of fat in major blood vessels, such as the aorta. A recent study from Hertfordshire in England showed low birth-weight babies, babies not doubling their birth-weight within 12 months and/or those who were breastfed beyond 12 months had much higher rates of vascular disease in later life. The theory behind this is that malnutrition for a foetus or during the first year of life leads to maldeveloped blood vessels that take up fat easily from an early stage. Interestingly, until five to 10 years ago, there was a significant amount of trans fatty acids in baby food, along with processed carbohydrates. This may have also contributed to the higher rates of coronary artery disease in those people considered malnourished as babies in the study.

Every piece of garbage that goes into the body in the form of synthetic food, exposure to passive smoking, or via the numerous environmental poisons leads to the membranes of our cells becoming progressively clogged with toxins. One of the first membranes to be damaged and subsequently destroyed is the membrane of the endothelial cell.

The endothelial cell lines every blood vessel in the body and is the first port of call for the nutrients in the bloodstream. Toxins damage the endothelial cell, thus allowing altered or oxidised cholesterol to travel easily across the damaged cell and into the subendothelial layer between the inner lining (known as the intima) and the muscle lining (known as the media). This is where the fatty plaque begins. It is, therefore, not the cholesterol itself, but the combination of the chemically based, free-radical attacks on the endothelium and the clogging of membranes with trans fatty acids that allows the altered sugar, protein and fat to form together into a sticky, fatty substance that becomes fatty plaque.

This process can occur anywhere between early childhood to late teens and then slowly builds up over decades—especially in arteries such as the coronary arteries, the carotid arteries leading to the brain, the aorta (the major blood vessel coming off the heart) and the blood vessels to the legs. In reality, all blood vessels are affected by this process to varying degrees.

If you asked most people, 'What happens during a heart attack?' they would tell you it is a progressive, slow blockage of an artery caused by cholesterol. This is not the case, it is a progressive swelling of the wall of an artery caused by the build-up of fat and altered or oxidised choles-terol; along with a chronic inflammatory response by the body and the subsequent deposition of calcium to try to strengthen a fatty plaque. If the plaques have a very large amount of fat, known as the lipid core, this combined with a thin cap over the top allows them to break down very easily. The calcium grows into the plaque as a reparative response by the body, attempting to act like a scaffold to strengthen the plaque and prevent it from breaking down.

As the wall of an artery swells with fat, the body maintains the internal channel for as long as possible. Therefore, a preventative screen for heart disease with tests such as stress tests or even angiograms has no real value. You can have one of these tests and be told everything is normal, nothing to worry about but a day later, a week later or a few months later, a large fatty plaque from one of your arteries ruptures. This certainly would not have been predicted by either of these tests.

This is the value of calcium scoring, which detects fatty plaques long before they have ruptured. With some of the newer machines, such as the multi-slice helical machine, earlier plaques without calcium can be detected.

The process of atherosclerosis is occurring in almost everyone living in Western society. The real issue is, at what rate is the fat being deposited? People with multiple major risk factors for coronary disease tend to have an accelerated rate of deposition of fat. A percentage of people with atherosclerosis will carry it with them to their death, perhaps at the ripe old age of 95. Just because atherosclerosis is present, it does *not* mean you will definitely have a heart attack. In the same way, just because you have high cholesterol, it does not necessarily mean you will have significant atherosclerosis either.

My dear, sweet mother in her mid-seventies had a total cholesterol reading of 9 millimoles per litre. Fortunately, she had an HDL level of 3 millimole per litre. Her doctor was keen for her to take a strong cholesterol-lowering agent. My response was, 'Before we do so, let's check her coronary arteries with the CT scanner.' Her score was zero and, in her case, the cholesterol was not spilling into her arteries to cause significant fatty plaques. She did not require cholesterol-lowering drugs.

No-one is really sure what event will precipitate a rupture of a plaque, but without doubt for a person with significant atherosclerosis, an acute life stress may be a major precipitant. I have seen quite a number of patients for whom symptoms came on after unusual physical activity. An overweight man running for the bus can put a strain on a fatty plaque causing it to rupture, leading to a subsequent blockage within the artery.

If you imagine a fatty plaque in an artery is like a pimple, instead of the plaque rupturing externally, it ruptures internally into the channel. Because there is a raw surface over the rupture, blood travels into the fatty plaque swelling the plaque. As the plaque swells, the ruptured site increases so the body forms a clot over this rupture, attempting to reduce swelling. The problem is that when the clot forms, it often causes a significant blockage within the channel and a subsequent heart attack. If the artery is blocked completely, the blood flow to this particular part of the heart muscle is impaired and can subsequently die and scar over. This is the process known as a heart attack, myocardial infarction, or coronary occlusion.

If there are smaller ruptures within the artery, and these ruptures are multiple, then blockages can build up over time within the arterial system, especially in the heart, and cause a lack of oxygen to the heart muscle without actually causing a heart attack. This can manifest as angina, which is a pain in the chest when you walk up a hill or become stressed. At times this lack of oxygen to the heart muscle can occur without any symptoms. If it is silent, this can be a real concern as the person does not know they have the underlying problem.

Although I believe cholesterol is an important component of athero-sclerosis, I am not convinced it is the primary cause. As I have argued, I feel it is the combination of free-radical attack and cell membrane damage from the accumulation of synthetic fats that allows these sticky, gluggy combinations of fat, sugar and protein to form the fatty plaques within the wall. I am not suggesting the cholesterol issue is purely a marker without any real part to play in the generation of heart disease, but I do not believe it is the major issue.

What pushes our cholesterol up in the first place? Certain types of fat—especially trans fatty acids, and to a lesser extent saturated fat—cause an elevation in LDL or 'bad' cholesterol, the most concerning part of the cholesterol molecule. To put it simply, the bad cholesterol mole-cule LDL is made of two components: one small and dense, the other large and buoyant. Because of the size of the large, buoyant proportion, it is not as oxidisable and it is harder for this part of the molecule to penetrate a damaged endothelium and set up its home in part of the fatty plaque. The small, dense LDL cholesterol is very easily oxidised by free radicals and thus escapes across the damaged cell wall to become part of the fatty plaque.

The concept of small, dense LDL cholesterol was first researched in Berkeley, California, by Dr Ron Krauss and Dr Robert Serpico, who had done some extraordinary work demonstrating the importance of small, dense LDL cholesterol as a major factor in the generation of heart disease. (One of the problems for people living outside the United States is that this measurement of cholesterol sub-fractions is not available.) The team at Berkeley estimated that around 50 per cent of heart disease is directly related to people with excessive amounts of small, dense LDL cholesterol in their bloodstream. The classic cholesterol profile for small, dense LDL cholesterol is a normal or minor elevation in cholesterol, a moderate elevation in triglyceride levels and a low HDL (or 'good' cholesterol) level. Unfortunately, around 30 per cent of people carrying small, dense LDL cholesterol have totally normal fat profiles.

The other interesting study performed in Dr Krauss' lab involved varying the fat intake for people with either a predominance of small, dense LDL or a predominance of large, buoyant LDL and seeing what effect these different diets had on the size of their LDL particle. Bear with me . . . this is very important, and fascinating! Around 240 healthy, non-smoking men consumed a high-fat diet (40 to 46 per cent of dietary fat); about 180 of them developed large, buoyant LDL cholesterol while the other 60 had small, dense LDL. Professor Krauss called the large, buoyant LDL 'pattern A' and the small, dense one 'pattern B'.

The real surprise came when all the men were switched to a reduced 20–24 per cent fat diet: 60 of the pattern-A men now became pattern B. An even greater shock came when 40 of the remaining pattern-A men were given a 10 per cent fat, high-carbohydrate diet. Twelve of these 40 men converted to pattern B.

This study clearly demonstrated that lowering the fat content of the diet could actually cause harm rather than do good. It also appears that the lower the fat content and the higher the carbohydrate content, the greater the risk of converting to the more dangerous pattern B.

We could conclude from this that it is the reduction in fat that is dangerous, but I believe it is the combination of fat reduction and the rise in the carbohydrate level that causes this harmful lipid profile. The reduction in fat strips the normal fat out of the membranes in the body and the rise in carbohydrates contributes to an increase in the triglyceride level and a reduction in the HDL (good) cholesterol. All of these changes can have harmful effects in the long term for most people. In my opinion, we need a reasonable proportion of fat to maintain a healthy overall lipid profile.

Life habits and cholesterols

I consult many patients who are horrified when their cholesterols are elevated. Often they will tell me they have been consuming a healthy diet for the past six months. What they fail to take into account is the very unhealthy diet they had for perhaps 60 years prior to this. The longer you abuse your body with poor eating habits, no exercise, cigarette smoking or other, illegal drugs and excessive alcohol, the more disordered your metabolism will become. This cannot always be completely reversed.

Excessive amounts of stress on the body can have varying effects on cholesterol. People who tend to be under chronic stress can push their cholesterol to high levels.

One of my patients, Daphne, has had bypass surgery and has always battled with her cholesterol level. I put her on an achievable but enjoyable lifestyle program along with two cholesterol-lowering drugs. Usually we achieve reasonable control of her cholesterol. Recently, Daphne had a prolonged holiday with friends and when she returned, she stated she'd had one of the best times of her life. We re-checked her cholesterol levels: they were the lowest they had ever been. Was this a coincidence or did the lack of stress and the enjoyment of the holiday contribute to the low level?

Interestingly, when someone suffers an acute heart attack or has bypass surgery, their cholesterol levels also tend to plummet. Therefore, it is important not to rely too much on cholesterol levels taken around the time of these events; it is better to re-check the level when the person has achieved a more steady state.

There is a definite association between weight and heart disease but the direct relationship to cholesterol is not as strong. Often patients who are carrying excessive amounts of weight have more the insulin-resistant profile, known as the dyslipidaemic profile, characterised by a slight elevation in cholesterol but a more pronounced elevation in triglycerides and a low HDL cholesterol.

There is no doubt that metabolism, which is the general process in the body driving our cells, varies between individuals. I have seen husband and wife allegedly eating the same food, and the husband has an enormously high cholesterol while the wife has a normal cholesterol level, and vice versa. There is no doubt that dietary habits have an effect on cholesterol levels, but this will only contribute around 25 per cent of the cholesterol level; the other 75 per cent comes from inherent metabolism.

Metabolism isn't just what you have inherited; it is also a combination of your life history, your lifelong living habits and the stresses and strains you are suffering at the time. For example, you can markedly change your metabolism by a period of poor eating and heavy drinking. Unfortunately, the system is more geared to sin than it is to penance and it takes the body time to recover.

I am always somewhat amused by the person who says, 'But Doctor, I only drink once a week.' If you avoid alcohol through the week then decide to consume your quota in one night, you are overloading your liver and it might take four to five days to recover. By that time, it's coming around to the next Saturday night when the abuse starts again. Thus, under these circumstances, for most of the week your major metabolic organ (i.e. your liver) is not functioning properly. Therefore you cannot hope to cope with any type of synthetic food load that is presented to your body.

There is also no doubt that some people are cursed with lousy genetics. No matter what wonderful and laudable lifestyle program they follow, their cholesterol will still be through the roof and they may develop premature vascular disease.

One of the most important principles I am trying to impart here, however, is not to be totally obsessed with cholesterol levels. As I have stated, the cholesterol profile is only one aspect of fat metabolism. Often it is far more concerning to me to see an elevation in triglycerides, which usually goes with a low HDL cholesterol, signifying the presence of the small, dense LDL cholesterol profile. If you think of oxidised LDL as the fat that easily travels into the wall of the artery, you should also think of a low HDL cholesterol as the stuff that sucks the fat out of the arteries. Therefore, the higher the HDL cholesterol, the less chance you have of fat travelling into the arteries in the first place, all other factors considered. Mind you, having a high HDL cholesterol is not a 100 per cent guarantee of longevity.

Case study: Eileen—In the days before measured lipoprotein(a) I had a patient who was a very youthful-looking 60-year-old woman. Eileen had a total cholesterol of 8 millimoles per litre and an HDL of 4. This was the highest HDL I had ever seen. Eileen's father had died in his fifties of a heart attack. I foolishly reassured Eileen that because her HDL was so high I was confident she would not have a heart attack. We had tried to lower her cholesterol with the agents available at the time (this was in the era before statins) and these pills either caused side effects or were ineffective. Eileen then said to me, 'I would prefer to have no pills at all and just follow a healthy diet.' I was quite comfortable in reassuring her that because of her high HDL she should have no problems at all. You can then imagine my shock and horror when Eileen's husband rang me to inform me that Eileen had died suddenly while on holiday at the age of 64. These days, with CT scanning of the coronary arteries and more advanced cardiac pathology, such as the measurement of lipoprotein(a), I would've detected her obvious significant atherosclerosis and been able to treat her problem.

There is strong evidence to suggest that the cholesterol–HDL ratio is a better marker for your risk for heart disease than the total cholesterol level. This very simple method of taking the total cholesterol and dividing it by the HDL gives a ratio. A concerning ratio is greater than 5. A preferable ratio is less than 3.5, and an extremely low-risk ratio is less than 2.5.

NATURAL WAYS TO INCREASE HDL (GOOD) CHOLESTEROL

These are the natural ways to increase HDL cholesterol, but there are other methods, which will be discussed later in the chapter.

• Weight loss.
• Regular physical exercise.

- Low-dose alcohol consumption: The consumption of two standard drinks per day has been shown to cause a modest increase in HDL cholesterol. There is, however, no doubt that if you go beyond the two standard glasses per day, you will affect liver metabolism, which will have the reverse effect on HDL cholesterol by increasing your triglycerides.
- Quitting smoking: Cigarette smokers generally have lower HDL cholesterols and the simple act of stopping smoking can restore the HDL to normal.
- Following a diet high in good fats: This will also tend to elevate HDL cholesterol.

Triglycerides

I keep bandying around the term triglycerides and you may be wondering what on earth these are and why are they important. Triglycerides have always been cholesterol's poorer cousin and have often been ignored. They are, in fact, the major by-product of dietary fat. When you consume a fatty meal, the fat is partially digested by bile and then absorbed into the body in large substances known as chylomicrons. When the chylomicrons are presented to the liver, triglycerides are extracted. Excessive triglycerides in the bloodstream, either straight after a meal or during the fasting state, can deliver more fat to LDL (bad) cholesterol and have an effect on reducing HDL (good) cholesterol.

It is, therefore, very important for doctors to carefully examine the entire profile and not to ignore even modest elevations in triglycerides. Elevated triglycerides are very common in:

1. overweight people
2. people with liver disease, especially alcohol-related
3. diabetics
4. those with an underactive thyroid
5. genetic triglyceride abnormalities.

When looking at the cholesterol profile, I suggest aiming for the following levels:

	No evidence of vascular disease	Proven vascular disease
Total cholesterol	Less than 5	Less than 4
LDL (bad) cholesterol	Less than 3	Less than 2
HDL (good) cholesterol	Greater than 1.3	Greater than 1.3
Triglycerides	Less than 1.5	Less than 1.5
Cholesterol–HDL ratio	Less than 3.5	Less than 2.5

The five-point approach to cholesterol management

You're wandering through the local mall and there's a mobile van offering a rapid health assessment. They check your blood pressure, do a pin-prick cholesterol and blood sugar test, measure your height and weight, rapidly give you the results . . . and often worry the life out of you. If your cholesterol is elevated, should you be rushing off to your local doctor demanding the latest and greatest pills? Should you be contacting your lawyer to get your will in order?

1. DON'T PANIC

A sobering but true statement is that tests can be wrong. Pin-prick finger cholesterol tests are notoriously inaccurate. I well remember the case of a truck driver who had his cholesterol checked this way and was told his cholesterol level was 4.8 and there was nothing to worry about. Two months later he had a heart attack. When his cholesterol was checked with a conventional blood test, his level was 7. I am not suggesting that all finger-prick cholesterols are completely inaccurate, but it is important to realise this could be the case.

The other important reliability aspect is the inter-lab variability. A very telling case concerns a man who attended my clinic with a cholesterol level of 7.1 from one laboratory, with a triglyceride level of 3.6. At my clinic one week later, his cholesterol was 5.1. I sent this information to his general practitioner, who then sent him to yet another laboratory, where his cholesterol level came back as 7.2. We now had three readings over the space of a few weeks—two of which were high and my reading which was low. On the strength of numbers, we were wrong. The patient, not wanting to commence cholesterol-lowering agents, came back to my lab to have another check. We took his blood again and sent it to two different laboratories. His cholesterol level was 5.2 on both readings. We now had four levels of around 5.1 and 5.2, and two levels in their 7s. I could then confidently state that the other two laboratories were wrong and our readings were right.

I didn't see the patient for a further 12 months until he returned for a further assessment and cholesterol check. His cholesterol by my reading was 7.2 with a triglyceride of 3.4. I asked him whether he had changed his habits over the past 12 months, and he hadn't. The question then is, which readings were right and which readings were wrong?

On further questioning, it appeared that the night before the man had had a heavy Chinese meal and more alcohol than he normally consumed. He had also had a screaming argument with his son. On further examination this man did have a rather volatile personality and it is difficult to say with any degree of conviction as to whether he had a marked variability in his cholesterol readings based on his food, alcohol consumption, or psyche at the time of the readings.

2. GET A FULL ASSESSMENT

Cholesterol levels alone should never be treated—the person should be treated. It is not enough to simply have a knee-jerk reaction: 'Your cholesterol is high, therefore you need a pill.' The big question is, 'Is your cholesterol abnormality really harming *you*?' It is not your total cholesterol level alone, but your overall lipid profile (of which cholesterol is only one part), combined with an accurate assessment by your doctor as to how much that lipid profile is putting you at risk for a future vascular event.

Many people will maintain a high cholesterol throughout their life and never develop a cardiac problem. The real skill is to know which person is being affected by lipid abnormality. An assessment of risk is based on the following five points:

(i) Clinical evaluation: Regardless of all the flash tests now available to assess cardiac risk, the most valuable is for the doctor to ask the right questions and perform the right examination. The greatest risk for heart disease is having had heart disease in the past. Therefore, if you have had a documented heart attack, a stent, or coronary artery bypass grafting or some other manifestation of vascular disease such as a stroke, aneurysm or blockages in your legs, you require aggressive treatment of your cholesterol, as one component in your risk-factor management.

(ii) Cigarette smoking, high blood pressure or a family history of vascular disease: These factors put you at much higher risk for a cardiac event in the future and, therefore, add to the justification of intensive management of your lipid abnormalities. On a more positive note, an equivocal rise in cholesterol with no evidence of risks for heart disease suggests you may be able to wait to commence cholesterol-lowering treatment. If someone has a low blood pressure, is a non-smoker and has both parents still alive and well in their eighties, this implies that this person may have inherited genetics somewhat protective against heart disease, regardless of the overall cholesterol levels.

My bias is, of course, towards very aggressive risk-factor assessment, but I am very much against looking at isolated cholesterol levels. Even if your doctor decides that you do not require more sophisticated tests, such as CT scanning, you should at least have as a baseline assessment of your cholesterol values, a fasting cholesterol, triglyceride, HDL and blood sugar level. It is my strong feeling that males over 40 and females over 50 should have a more extensive work up than just these blood tests.

(iii) Cardiac risk: The real question is, how much of the cholesterol and fat in your body is ending up in the blood vessels, causing atheroscleros? Only 50 per cent of heart disease can be explained by high cholesterol, cigarette smoking and high blood pressure. The other 50 per cent is due to a whole host of abnormalities, such as the newer risk factors that have only been highlighted in the past 10 years or so. It is my firm opinion that lipoprotein(a), homocysteine and highly sensitive C-reactive protein should also be performed as part of this routine screen.

High-speed CT scanning of the heart is also central to estimating someone's true risk for heart disease. With the increasing evidence showing the highly accurate predictive value of CT scanning, most of its critics have been silenced over the past few years. The CT scan is non-invasive. It takes pictures using minimal doses of irradiation (somewhere between four and five times a chest X-ray), looking for calcium and fat in the coronary arteries. The newer machines can not only calculate the amount of calcium in the arteries, but also see fatty plaques without calcium.

The amount of calcium is closely related to the amount of fat in the arteries. Calcium itself is not the problem, but if there is calcium, there is certainly fat in the area, and it is the fat that may rupture to cause a heart attack. From all the most recent studies, there is clear evidence that the more calcium and fat in your arteries, the higher your risk for a heart attack or sudden cardiac death.

It is, therefore, my feeling that if you have a zero or very low calcium score, with all other risk factors and clinical assessment considered, there is not much point in considering cholesterol-lowering pills at this stage. If your score is high, however, I believe it is important that your entire profile is managed aggressively.

The score can be presented in two ways:
(a) Absolute calcium score
    Zero   very limited risk for heart attack over 10 years
    1–100   mild fat build-up in the arteries—low coronary risk

101–400   moderate fat content in arteries—moderate risk

Greater   large fat load in arteries—high risk
than 400

(b) Percentile ranking

Recent studies have shown that percentile ranking is a more accurate way of assessing risk. If you line up 100 people of the same sex and age and perform calcium scores, it is those people in the greater-than-50th percentile that have the highest risk. For example, approximately 40 per cent of 50-year-old males may have a zero score and the remaining 60 per cent will have a score anywhere from 1 up to the thousands. If one of the men had a score of 30 he might be in the top 75th percentile ranking, therefore, at a high risk of a cardiac event despite the relatively low score. A 70-year-old male with a score of 150 might, however, be in the 30th percentile ranking —therefore, at low risk. The reason for the variation is the older the person is, the more likelihood of some degree of atherosclerosis, and as the arteries age they also tend to calcify more and are therefore less likely to break down to cause a heart attack. So, looking at the absolute score is not always the best approach, but combining the absolute score and percentile ranking gives a much better overall assessment of risk.

(iv) Follow-up: One of the most important aspects of any long-term preventative strategy is follow-up. There is no point performing all these high-powered assessments, giving all this good information and possibly commencing a medication strategy without ensuring that the person is performing well and achieving the set targets.

I believe that within six to 12 weeks of commencing any new preventative strategy involving cholesterol modification, it is important to repeat the tests for cholesterol values. If the person is taking a cholesterol-lowering pill, I would routinely order cholesterol, triglyceride, HDL, ALT (liver enzyme) and CPK (muscle enzyme) levels, along with a blood sugar and uric acid level. I'm always disappointed when my patients return to their doctor and the doctor omits some of these tests. I believe they should be performed routinely on a regular basis. After you have been stabilised on the program, the tests should be performed every six to 12 months, based on your doctor's recommendations.

If I detect calcium scores above 200, or when a person is in the greater-than-75th percentile or suffering symptoms suggestive of heart problems, I would then progress to stress echocardiography. Stress testing has been the cornerstone of non-invasive assessment of heart disease for many years but I believe a stress test without some form of imaging is now outmoded, apart from for a limited group of people. It is my preference to perform stress echocardiography because there is no radiation involved, it takes less of the patient's time, it costs the community and the medical system around half that of a stress nuclear scan and is just as accurate.

The gold standard for the diagnosis of blockages in the coronary arteries, however, is coronary angiography. Coronary angiography is a very safe test in expert hands, but still requires invasion into the body. The artery is entered with a needle either in the groin or the arm. Catheters are placed in the heart and dye is flushed down the arteries, providing an accurate picture of the arteries.

CT scanning of the coronary arteries is not a replacement for coronary angiography because it looks at a totally different aspect of the artery. CT scanning looks at the wall of the artery and, therefore, detects atherosclerosis long before a blockage would occur. If there is evidence that the heart has a significant lack of oxygen to put the muscle under stress on the combination of CT scanning and stress echocardiography, there is then good justification to perform a coronary angiogram.

Case study: Bernard—After a CT scan Bernard told me he was not suffering pain, but every time he walked beyond a gentle stroll he noticed an unusual feeling in his chest. The 'unusual feeling' and his extremely high calcium score, along with the presence of diabetes, high blood pressure and moderate obesity, suggested to me that this man had significant blockages in his arteries. (I must state, it wouldn't have taken Einstein to figure this one out!)

I immediately admitted him to our local hospital, where a coronary angiogram demonstrated severe triple vessel blockages in his arteries. He had urgent coronary artery bypass surgery. Since that time, he has completely changed his lifestyle, achieved excellent diabetic and cholesterol control, along with exquisite blood pressure control and I am confident these strategies are keeping him very well.

One area of controversy is monitoring the progression of atherosclerosis with CT scanning. There is an increasing amount of work in the United States showing great value in monitoring. The preliminary work from my laboratory suggests it is better to wait two years before a repeat scan and in some cases, three to five years is sufficient. Once the stabilisation or reversal of atherosclerosis is achieved, I am not sure there is much point performing further scans—apart from patient reassurance within five to ten years' time to demonstrate the disease is being controlled.

(v) Target values: There is no point commencing cholesterol-lowering therapy unless you are confident it is achieving its aims. If you start a lifestyle strategy and after three to six months it makes no difference whatsoever to your cholesterol level, and you have been deemed at high risk for a future cardiac event, this is strong indication that you need to start on a cholesterol-lowering pill. The situation is somewhat analogous to treating blood pressure. If you commence a blood pressure-lowering pill and your blood pressure does not come down, then your doctor has to re-think treatment strategies. This is why it is so important to aim for target values and ensure you achieve values very close to these levels.

3. DRUGS ARE NOT SUFFICIENT ON THEIR OWN

Every month I receive, as part of my normal continuing medical education, a copy of the two world premier journals in cardiology: the *Journal of the American College of Cardiology* and *Circulation*. On the back of one of these journals was an advertisement I thought was one of the greatest scandals in cardiology. The ad read in big letters, 'When diet and exercise fail, meet yet another candidate for [drug X]', which happened to be a common cholesterol-lowering pill.

What irritated me was the notion that diet and exercise fail.

Diet and exercise *never* fail! Lifestyle interventions *never* fail! I would like to make these emphatic statements because in this particular case it is true. There is no doubt that there are people for whom diet, exercise or other lifestyle interventions will not be enough, but they never *fail!* In fact, I would like to make the point that cholesterol-lowering drugs *without* diet and exercise really have little value. If combined with a lifestyle program, however, I believe the cholesterol-lowering drugs become very powerful.

There is a distorted concept that cholesterol-lowering pills mean you can loosen your diet somewhat. I have heard of many people ingesting a large trans fatty acid, processed carbohydrate-laden diet then swallowing a couple of extra cholesterol-lowering pills to cover the possible mayhem created by this behaviour. What this person doesn't realise is that the effect of acute bad fat and carbohydrate loads on the body are not just manifested through a high cholesterol. A study where people were fed a breakfast from a popular takeaway food outlet and had their endothelial function—or the ability of their arteries to dilate when they exercised—showed a reduced ability of the arteries' normal dilating by around 50 per cent. Having this sort of acute or chronic diet also thickens the blood markedly, regardless of the cholesterol level. Please, if you take nothing else from this chapter, realise pills are not a substitute for a healthy lifestyle!

If you do have evidence of significant atherosclerosis, or have already had a cardiac problem, a healthy lifestyle will probably not be enough. There is no doubt that lifestyle intervention will give you a very good start, but if you are already very advanced in your cardiac career, you need more help with very aggressive cholesterol-lowering drugs.

4. MULTIPLE THERAPY

Managing cholesterol should be analogous to managing blood pressure. Some people require one pill, some people require two pills, and unfortunately, some people may require three or four pills. As far as cardiac prevention goes, there are five types of responses from patients to the intervention or treatment offered by doctors.

The first and most interesting one is where the person is told they have a problem and, either due to denial or a differing opinion by another member of the profession, they are lost in the system and don't follow up. So I really don't know what happens with them.

Case study: Lost soul—A patient at my clinic had a CT scan score of 350. This placed him at a moderate risk for future atherosclerotic events. It was our advice he should have a stress echocardiogram or a stress nuclear scan to determine whether there was any evidence of blockages in his arteries. His general practitioner referred him to a local cardiologist who performed a stress nuclear scan, which was completely normal. The cardiologist then informed him that his heart was totally normal and the information he'd been given at our clinic was 'rubbish'— he should demand his money back.

This shows complete ignorance of what CT scanning is trying to demonstrate. CT scanning gives a very accurate assessment of the degree of fat and calcium in the wall of the arteries. This man clearly had coronary artery disease, but it was not as yet causing a blockage in his arteries and, therefore, he did not as yet have heart trouble. I totally agree with the cardiologist, the man's heart was normal, but, I was concerned about his future risk for developing a heart problem. He had moderately advanced atherosclerosis and, therefore, required global treatment for his atherosclerotic risk.

The second type of response is where the person has a CT scan, accepts the results, doesn't attempt to change his lifestyle but will take medication. When he returns for reassessment and the results have clearly deteriorated, he is surprised and somewhat disappointed. Only a fool believes something will change when he continues behaving the way he has always behaved. Unless a person alters their lifestyle and, possibly, takes supplemental medications and antioxidants, nothing is going to change in their arteries. I see this in people who have not changed their eating habits or their exercise habits—they put their fat gut on my table and say, 'Doc, it appears these cholesterol-lowering pills aren't working.'

The third type concerns patients who only require lifestyle and anti-oxidant treatment.

Case study: Successfully working—One of the bosses of a multinational food company that produces a cholesterol-lowering margarine scored 1400 on the CT scanner. His cholesterol was 6.5, HDL 1.2, and triglycerides 2.5. I performed a stress echocardiogram, which was basically normal, suggesting he did not require a coronary angiogram or further invasive treatment. He did, however, require aggressive management of his athero-sclerosis. I suggested he make significant lifestyle changes and also started him on a cholesterol-lowering pill because of the magni-tude of his atherosclerosis.

I did not hear from him for two years, then he returned for a follow-up CT scan. His cholesterol had dropped to 4.6, he had lost significant weight with a markedly improved diet and exercise program, but he had made the decision not to take the cholesterol-lowering pill. When I repeated the CT scan his score had dropped to 800 with a significant improvement in his arteries. He had used the cholesterol-lowering margarines his company made and this, combined with marked lifestyle change, had, in his case, caused a major reduction in his atherosclerotic disease.

The fourth group involves patients who need a cholesterol-lowering drug. These people respond to lifestyle changes, antioxidants, low-dose Aspirin and a single cholesterol-lowering drug. They follow through and I have had numerous people in this group return for repeat CTs and show great stabilisation in their arteries—in many cases, a reversal. Professor Callister's group from Nashville have also demonstrated with CT scanning of the coronaries that the combination of lifestyle and cholesterol-lowering therapy is very beneficial in this setting.

Unfortunately those in the fifth group require aggressive lifestyle modification, low-dose Aspirin and antioxidant therapy, combined with management of their blood pressure and at least double cholesterol-lowering treatment. If they stick with it they can achieve success. The cold, hard facts of the matter are that people with stable coronary artery disease have a 2 per cent yearly death rate.

DOUBLE OR NOTHING?

Professor Greg Brown from Seattle performed a study of men with proven heart disease on a coronary angiogram over five years and placed them on varying combinations of cholesterol-lowering agents. He achieved the best reversal of heart disease by using a combination of one of the statin drugs (see later in the chapter) and nicotinic acid (Niacin, a high dose of Vitamin B3).

Seventy of those in the study, having achieved such a wonderful response, said to Professor Brown, 'We feel so well on this combination we would really like to continue on these drugs and stay under your care.' Brown then followed these 70 men for a further five years. At the end there should have been around 14 deaths but, remarkably, there were none. In fact, of the 70 patients only one suffered a minor heart attack over the full 10-year period. This is almost unheard of in a group of people with quite severe

> coronary artery disease. It is my feeling that if I had significant atherosclerosis—especially if I had already suffered a heart attack or had undergone bypass surgery—I would be taking double cholesterol-lowering therapy.

5. CHOLESTEROL-LOWERING THERAPY IS FOR LIFE

I know some patients who suffer the misconception that once the cholesterol has been brought back to normal they can stop taking the pill. If your cholesterol is contributing to your significant atherosclerosis, a course of therapy will control your cholesterol only for the time you are taking this medication. Therefore, you must stay on this treatment for the rest of your life, or until some better therapy has been discovered. Each year new agents are being tested and I am confident that as scientific research continues, the drugs involved will have less side effects and more power to control the overall lipid profile. There are quite a few new drugs on the horizon that are showing great promise in early testing.

One of the problems with being on lifelong therapy is the potential for side effects. (The major side effects of the cholesterol-lowering drugs will be discussed in the next section.) And no-one can guarantee that cholesterol-lowering pills, either alone or in combination, are safe over a prolonged period of time. If you are only in your thirties or forties and your doctor suggests you should start taking a pill on a lifelong basis, you may be taking this pill for the next 30 to 40 years. The newer cholesterol-lowering drugs have only been available for 10 to 15 years. Unfortunately, there have been far too many medications or substances that had been deemed to be harmless or even good for you in some way, but after 20 to 25 years they have been shown to create a problem.

In the '50s and '60s, there was a drug known as Stilboestrol, which was used to avert premature labour in pregnant women. Twenty years later, it was found that the daughters of the women who used Stilboestrol had a higher rate of cervical cancer. Fifteen to 20 years after the treatment for cancer with chemotherapy, there is a high rate of secondary tumours. These two incidences show that there is a basic problem when you expose your body to an unnatural chemical. I would, however, not just single out drugs in this respect. We expose ourselves to unnatural chemicals almost every moment of the day, and none of us can really be sure as to the long-term effects of those chemicals.

Regarding the treatment of cholesterol, there is much debate in the scientific world as to the effect on cholesterol metabolism. There is a school of thought that suggests that lowering the cholesterol too much can alter membrane function—especially in the brain. One such opinion is that excessive lowering of cholesterol can lead to depression and problems with thinking. This is certainly not the case in cultures with lifelong low cholesterol rates, possibly because their bodies are adapted to having these cholesterol levels.

When you bring in any form of metabolic change, there is the potential for risk. The rates of depression and cognitive problems may be related to the drop in cholesterol or, possibly, to a side effect of the drugs, or may even be a statistical aberration. It is my strong feeling, however, that if your cholesterol is high and you have significant atherosclerosis, then your vascular disease will kill you long before the treatment of your cholesterol will. In that setting it is therefore vital to use every trick in the book to control your cholesterol.

The most important aspect in the management of any chronic condition is to establish a firm relationship with a doctor you can trust and have regular follow-up assessments with this doctor. If you decide to stop taking the pills, it is very important you check with your doctor first, explaining the reasons why this is your wish. The stark reality for the medical profession is that in patients with a chronic problem, somewhere between 30 and 50 per cent no longer take the prescribed medications 12 months after starting on the drugs. I don't know how many intelligent and motivated people I have seen who have said, 'I ran out of the script and hadn't bothered to get a new script filled.' I then proceed to find the nearest brick wall and start banging my head against it.

Cholesterol-lowering treatments

If you have high cholesterol and are at high risk for heart disease you need to do something about it. There are two major approaches:

1. natural cholesterol-lowering strategies
2. pharmaceutical agents (drugs).

1. NATURAL CHOLESTEROL-LOWERING STRATEGIES

Let's get back to our old mate Hippocrates, and let food be our medicine. Following the principles of this book, the first and most important step on the way to achieving a better lipid or cholesterol profile is let food be your medicine. Simply put, we have the following:

(a) Avoid synthetic food—reduce trans fatty acids and processed carbohydrates.
(b) Increase your good fats—your essential fatty acids, especially the Omega-3 and Omega-6 fats and also mono-unsaturated fatty acids.
(c) Increase the antioxidant content of your diet.
(d) Consume good-quality proteins.
(e) Modify your ingestion of neutral foods, such as saturated fats and complex carbohydrates.

All of these points are covered in more detail in the nutrition sections of this book. Losing weight will also contribute to an improved lipid profile. A combination of calorie restriction and increased exercise is the most important formula for losing weight.

Regarding the natural supplements available to treat cholesterol, there are quite a few showing promise. The word 'supplement' fits perfectly in this situation—they are supplements to a healthy lifestyle and may also be used as supplements to a stronger pharmaceutical agent. The sensible use of combinations may also help reduce the dose of pharmaceuticals necessary to achieve target cholesterol levels.

Fish oil capsules: Low-dose fish oil capsules (i.e. 1000 mg daily) have been shown to cause a significant reduction in future cardiac events and sudden cardiac death in people with established heart disease. Low-dose fish oil capsules reduce heart disease by thinning the blood and improving membrane function. To have any sort of effect on your overall lipid profile you need to take at least six capsules a day. Many people cannot tolerate this amount of fish oil capsules, but a moderate dose of fish oil capsules daily may be of some benefit, especially to people with triglyceride problems.

Co-enzyme Q10: Co-enzyme Q10 has many powerful actions throughout the body. It is known in some circles as the cardiac antioxidant. In fact, it would probably be better known as the muscle antioxidant, which includes, of course, the cardiac muscle. The energy production site in cells is known as the mitochondria. Without a constant supply of energy our cells cannot function normally. The major energy supply of the body is known as adenosine triphosphate (ATP). Co-enzyme Q10 is an essential co-factor for the production of ATP. Although it was initially discovered in 1957, it is still not widely accepted by the medical profession as being important as a supplement.

As a cholesterol-lowering agent, it is weak, but it has a synergistic effect if used with the statin agents (lipitor, pravachol, zocor, mevacor, lescol, vastin, lipex, etc.), which lower cholesterol by blocking the HMG Co-A reductase enzyme. There is some theoretical evidence showing that when statins are used, the level of co-enzyme Q10 is depleted throughout the body, especially in the muscles. Muscle aches and pains and, rarely, severe muscle damage are consequences of long-term use of statins. In many cases, this can be reversed or at least reduced by the use of co-enzyme Q10 50 to 100 mg a day. If you decide to take co-enzyme Q10 with a statin, I suggest you take it at the same time.

Q10 AND HEART FAILURE

There have been well over 20 trials using co-enzyme Q10 in the treatment of heart failure. A minority of these trials showed no benefit. Some trials showed a reduction in symptoms and others improved survival using varying doses of co-enzyme Q10, between 30 and 200 mg per day. Co-enzyme Q10 has also been shown to be of value in treating angina and, because of its ability to act as an antioxidant, it has been found to reduce some of the complications of cardiac surgery if used for two to three months before the operation.

If you choose to use co-enzyme Q10, it is more effective when taken with Vitamin E. As a maintenance dose I would suggest at least 50 mg a day of co-enzyme Q10 taken with somewhere between 400 and 800 international units (iu) a day of Vitamin E.

Policosanol: This is a natural cholesterol-lowering agent derived from the waxy portion of sugar cane. There have been over 19 studies involving around 30 000 patients demonstrating its benefit. It had a very strong safety profile with limited side effects in all of the studies. Statin agents work by blocking the HMG Co-A reductase enzymes. Policosanol is a modulator of this enzyme, so in a way it can be seen as a weak 'natural' statin agent. The usual dose of Policosanol is somewhere between 5 and 10 mg taken with the evening meal. It has an ability to lower LDL and total cholesterol when compared with a low dose of a statin agent. I believe there are three groups of people who would benefit from considering policosanol therapy. Those with:

(i)   an inability to take stronger pharmaceutical agents due to side effects;
(ii) mild to moderate increase in cholesterol deemed to be at mild to moderate risk by other tests such as CT scanning of the coronaries; and
(iii) an aversion to taking stronger pharmaceutical agents.

The downside of using Policosanol on a long-term basis is the expense: in Australia, Policosanol costs around $40 per month.

Red clover: Red clover is one of the isoflavone products and, in a dose of 40 mg daily, has been shown to cause a slight reduction in cholesterol, but in one particular study it caused a 28 per cent increase in HDL cholesterol. Because of all the other benefits of taking isoflavones, especially in peri-menopausal women, it may be worth considering supplementing with one of these products. It is important to realise that the significant HDL-raising ability has only been demonstrated in isoflavones from the red clover source.

B Group vitamins: Vitamin B3 (niacin) and, to a lesser extent, Vitamin B5 (pantothenic acid), have been found to be useful in the treatment of cholesterol abnormalities. Vitamin B3 in pharmacologic doses really should be considered in the pharmaceutical group (I'll discuss this in more detail in the next section).

Regarding Vitamin B5, a dose of around 900 mg a day has been shown to not only lower cholesterol but also to increase HDL.

2. PHARMACEUTICAL AGENTS
In Western society, cholesterol-lowering agents are among the most commonly prescribed drugs. Not all cholesterol-lowering drugs are created equal and different cholesterol-lowering drugs have different effects on the overall lipid profile. On numerous occasions, I've seen patients able to reverse their atherosclerosis and also reverse the lack of oxygen to their heart muscle with a combination of lifestyle changes and the use of cholesterol-lowering pills.

There are various drugs available.

Bile acid binding agents: There are two agents available on the market: cholestyramine and colestipol. Both are effective in lowering LDL (bad) cholesterol, and are available in a powder form that has to be mixed with juice. The suggested dose is four sachets per day, but I have a small number of people who can achieve excellent cholesterol lowering with one sachet a day—especially when combined with a statin. If either of these agents is to be used, it is vital to remember that no other medication should be taken for around two hours either side of taking one of these sachets. What happens is these agents will bind the drugs in the gut and they will not be absorbed. Therefore, if you are to use a bile acid binding agent, I suggest you take it in the morning and take your cholesterol-lowering agent, such as a statin, in the evening.

The major side effects of the bile acid binding agents are related to the gastrointestinal tract. A significant number of people taking these agents, especially at the higher doses, spend a great portion of their time in the bathroom with abdominal pain, bloating, constipation or diahorrea.

Nicotinic Acid: Also known as Vitamin B3 or niacin, nicotinic acid is one of the oldest methods available for lowering cholesterol. It is not commonly used these days because of statins but Vitamin B3 is an essential and natural vitamin, and in pharmacologic doses it is an excellent cholesterol-lowering agent. The recommended daily allowance of niacin is 20 mg. This amount is easily achieved by eating some sort of fortified food, such as breakfast cereal, or consuming fruits and vegetables.

A deficiency of Vitamin B3 is known as pellagra, which causes an unusual form of dermatitis and early onset dementia. This is, of course, very rare in Western society and is now confined to the fine print of medical textbooks. Low doses of Vitamin B3 have absolutely no effect on cholesterol, nor does the related compound, nicotinamide. Many of my patients who cannot tolerate high doses of Vitamin B3 switch over to nicotinamide, falsely believing it will help lower their cholesterol.

There is no doubt that statin agents are the most effective in lowering LDL and total cholesterol levels, but as I have demonstrated throughout this book, it is not always the total cholesterol or LDL level that is the problem. In fact, only pravachol of all the statins has a significant benefit in lowering small, dense LDL cholesterol, which is of much greater concern than the total LDL level.

Nicotinic acid also significantly lowers triglyceride levels and small, dense LDL cholesterol, and is, in fact, the best agent to raise HDL cholesterol. Whereas statins and gemfibrozil can raise HDL cholesterol by somewhere between 10 and 15 per cent, nicotinic acid in doses greater than 1 gram a day can raise HDL cholesterol by up to 25–30 per cent.

The FATS trial (the Familial Atherosclerosis Therapy Study, performed by Professor Greg Brown from Seattle) showed that the use of a statin and nicotinic acid is the best combination to reverse coronary heart disease. These studies performed over a five-year period caused a

90 per cent reduction in cardiac events, which is in stark contrast to the 30 per cent reduction seen using statins alone. Well, you may ask, why aren't these things in the drinking water? The reason is, unfortunately, as with everything in life, there's no such thing as a free lunch. They are damned difficult to take.

If I gave you a 250 mg nicotinic acid tablet on an empty stomach, you'd go bright red. It's like someone running a blow torch up your back. You need to ease this medication gently into your system. It is my suggestion that you start with a quarter of a tablet twice a day right in the middle of a meal, gradually increasing this dosage over a few months to two tablets twice daily. It's a real hassle taking this agent, but with the obvious benefit in reversing heart disease, especially when used in combination with a statin, it is certainly worth the effort.

There are now slow-release preparations on the market but I would add some caution here. The earlier slow-release preparations showed a significant proportion of liver problems after long-term ingestion. With the newer slow-release preparations, liver problems have been abolished. A 2000 mg preparation in the United States has been very effective, and in Australia there is also a 500 mg tablet known as niacinol, with one to two taken twice daily. Although niacinol is effective and easy to take and has minimal side effects, it is much weaker than immediate-acting nicotinic acid, therefore it does not have the same benefits on the lipid profile.

Case study: Abe Peters—Abe Peters is 52 years old. At 49 he was jogging and noted a severe bout of chest pain when he ran. He ignored this, attributing it to the spicy Indian curry he'd had the night before. The next day, sitting in his office during a rather heated telephone conversation with a client, he noted the same tightness increasing in his chest, to the point of quite significant discomfort. The pain did not abate so Abe sensibly rang the ambulance and was immediately transported to a local hospital.

A coronary angiogram was performed and there was a total obstruction in the left anterior descending artery, the main artery in his heart. The cardiologist at the hospital inserted a stent across the artery, restoring the blood flow in the damaged area. Abe had a 40 per cent block in his right coronary artery and a 20 per cent blockage in the circumflex.

Following discharge from hospital, he started on a statin along with low-dose Aspirin and a new blood-thinning drug known as Clopidogrel. His doctor had also used an anti-anginal agent known as a beta blocker. His profile before commencing treatment revealed a total cholesterol of 6.6 millimoles per litre (mmol/L), triglycerides 3 mmol/L, HDL cholesterol 1 mmol/L. Abe, being a classic type-A person, commenced an ultra low-fat diet and initially lost 5 kilograms and was feeling very well.

After a few months, stresses returned to his life. His diet became less rigid and his cardiologist noted that his cholesterol was edging up slightly. Abe was given a higher dose of statin agents and his cholesterols were measured again. His total cholesterol was now 4.8 mmol/L, his triglycerides remained elevated at 2.9 mmol/L and his HDL 1.1 mmol/L.

Eighteen months later his chest pain recurred and, following an abnormal exercise test, it was decided to repeat his angiogram. The angiogram showed the stent in his anterior descending artery was partially reclosed to around 30 per cent but the lesion seen before in his right and circumflex arteries had now progressed to greater than 70 per cent. I suggested strongly that Abe undergo coronary artery bypass grafting.

The question you must ask in this situation is why his disease progressed despite what would be considered reasonable treatment for underlying coronary artery disease. The reason in Abe's case is what is known as the dyslipidaemic profile. The dyslipidaemic profile is a cholesterol abnormality occurring in around 50 per cent of cases of coronary artery disease. Although the total cholesterol is controlled, statin agents have little effect on small, dense LDL cholesterol, especially in people who are not adhering strictly to their diet. Abe's diet initially was quite acceptable, but as he slipped back into his normal habit of having a piece of cake or a muffin for morning tea, and not really pursuing his exercise program, his small, dense LDL cholesterol would have risen quite dramatically, despite the total reduction in cholesterol. This is clearly seen on his lipid profile with not much difference in the triglycerides and HDL, suggesting an ongoing problem from small, dense LDL. The fat still pours into the arteries and more aggressive treatment is needed.

It is important to stress that nicotinic acid is not a replacement for Cell Factor therapy. It is just part of the treatment and will certainly give added benefit. Another major benefit of nicotinic acid is its ability to lower lipoprotein(a). This is reduced by around 30 per cent by high-dose nicotinic acid.

Fibric acid derivatives: Around 25 to 30 years ago, a drug known as Atromid-S was released onto the market. This was supposed to be the new wonder drug for cholesterol lowering. While it had a reasonable effect on some aspects of the lipid profile, it was shown to cause side effects and there was a concern raised about its ability to contribute to gastrointestinal cancers and gall bladder disease. Since then, a few newer fibric acid derivatives have become available.

The most commonly prescribed agent is gemfibrozil. When it was released, a study known as the Helsinki Heart Study revealed a 36 per cent reduction in cardiovascular disease with the use of gemfibrozil. Headlines, however, came out announcing: 'Cholesterol-lowering drug causes suicide and violent death'. This is one of the bizarre aspects of medical reporting. When you examine this study carefully, there were 10 deaths from suicide or violence from the few thousand people in the study group who were taking gemfibrozil. There were only four deaths from the same causes in the control group. Strangely enough, when these deaths were examined more closely, five out of the 10 people allegedly taking gemfibrozil had stopped taking the drug before their death. In reality, then there were only five deaths from suicide or violence in people taking gemfibrozil, and nine deaths in this study in people who were not taking gemfibrozil. You could then come to the bizarre conclusion that gemfibrozil *prevented* murder and suicide. Of course, both of these conclusions are ridiculous.

There are some psychologists and psychiatrists who argue that lowering cholesterol levels indirectly affects the chemicals in the brain known as serotonin and catecholamines, making people more prone to depression, suicide and anti-social behaviour. This theory has not been proven but should certainly not be dismissed.

When the results from the Helsinki Heart Study and a similar study known as the PROCAM study were analysed, it was shown that there was a marked increase in heart attacks and sudden cardiac death in the patients with a cholesterol–HDL ratio greater than 5, and triglycerides greater than 2. Treatment with gemfibrozil in this group showed a 75 per cent reduction in cardiac events and death rates. This emphasises the point that we should streamline the treatment of our patients with cholesterol abnormalities and not specifically attempt to lower LDL cholesterol without analysing triglyceride and HDL.

Case study: Tony Sundin—Tony Sundin is 52 years old. He arrived at his local hospital with increasing chest pain and was found to have a major blockage in his right coronary artery requiring a coronary stent. When his blood was analysed, his total cholesterol was 6 mmol/L but his triglyceride level was 10 mmol/L and his HDL was 1. He was given Atorvastatin, one of the powerful statin agents, which brought his cholesterol down to 5 but his triglycerides remained at 10. He felt perfectly well, but when he came to me for a second opinion I realised Tony had a significant problem with combined hyerlipidaemia and not just a problem with LDL cholesterol. I cut back his 40 mg of Atorvastatin to 20, and added gemfibrozil in a dose of 600 mg twice a day.

Tony returned a month later, at which time I again measured his cholesterol, triglyceride, HDL, ALT and CPK levels, along with blood sugar. Tony was very diligent with his lifestyle and I was convinced that most of his cardiac problems were genetically based. He was thin and athletic but had been under considerable stress. His father had died a few years before following a major heart attack. When I reviewed his cholesterol levels, his total cholesterol had dropped to 4.5, his triglycerides were 1.3 and his HDL was also 1.3. This was a remarkable turnaround compared with his prior results. His liver and muscle enzymes and his blood sugar were entirely normal.

I believe there is an important place for fibric acid derivatives on the market and in fact, a new drug known as Fenofibrate is soon to be released on the Australian market and is already available in the United States.

Statins: The statins are the world champions in the cholesterol-lowering stakes and are very powerful agents in reducing total cholesterol and LDL levels. There have been five major studies of statin therapy demonstrating a 20 to 30 per cent reduction in heart attack, angina and the need for surgical intervention, along with a reduction in total death rates.

There are a variety of statins on the market and the decision about which agent is prescribed is really up to the individual doctor. The side-effect profile is very similar: muscle aches and pains and, rarely, severe destruction of the muscles known as rhabdomyolysis. Usually, when a person suffers muscle aches and pains with a statin, their CK levels (muscle enzyme levels) are elevated. The figures quoted are up to one in 20 people will suffer muscle aches and pains, but it is my suspicion that over the long term this figure is much higher. The aches and pains stop within a few days of stopping therapy and I have seen benefit from using co-enzyme Q10 in conjunction with a statin, to abolish or reduce this symptom.

Pravastatin is a water-soluble statin and also tends to have a lower side-effect profile. Pravastatin seems to have a better effect on small, dense LDL cholesterol and has been shown to have positive effects on other aspects of atherosclerosis, such as improved endothelial function and a reduction in 'blood thickness' by affecting clotting proteins and platelets.

There are many researchers in the field who believe that statins basically have similar actions and side effects. Some people believe that the more powerful the statin, the better the effect on the overall atherosclerotic process; whereas others hold that once you've achieved a certain level of cholesterol lowering, there is no added benefit beyond this.

In around 2–3 per cent of cases, the liver can also be affected. This is very simply assessed by routinely performing an ALT (liver enzyme test) every time the lipid levels are checked.

Statins should be used in almost all cases of people with proven vascular disease or significant atherosclerosis seen on CT scanning, but it is unacceptable for people to tolerate side effects. Severe muscle aches and pains are certainly a contraindication to continuing statin therapy. Statins have also been shown to affect concentration, increase depression, reduce libido and contribute to impotence. Although these side effects are not particularly common, they certainly do occur and should be reported if you are being affected.

Newer therapies: There are many new agents that will probably be released in the next few years. One that shows real promise is a drug known as Ezetimide (Zetia). This drug inhibits cholesterol absorption and, when recently tried with a large dose of a statin, was four times more effective in reducing LDL cholesterol than doubling the dose of the statin.

With the improved screening techniques for vascular disease and the greater awareness of the medical profession, and the public, of the more intricate aspects of lipid abnormalities, a more sensible approach for the management of people with these problems is now occurring. We need to lose the distorted concept that the solution to all of our ills is in a pill or potion, and realise that cholesterol abnormalities are just a part of the problem—not the entire cause for vascular disease.

An integrated approach involving sensible lifestyle, appropriate supplementation and cholesterol-lowering medications, when necessary, will afford the best long-term results. As with all medical problems, an open, long-term relationship with your doctor is the best solution.

HYPERTENSION

When we think of high blood pressure, we usually think of a prototype highly stressed individual, ranting and raving, red in the face, throwing things and hoping desperately they hit the target. Although people who exhibit this rather bizarre behaviour are more likely to push their blood pressure up, high blood pressure in almost all cases is a genetic/metabolic disease. If one of your parents or a first-degree relative has the condition then it's the sperm–ovum combo that has set up your genetic make-up, contributing to the problem. Of course, if you have a lousy life or a life that is stress after stress, then you will probably develop high blood pressure long before your identical twin that has sailed through life without any major traumas. But in the end, both of you will get it.

The strict definition of hypertension is 'elevated blood pressure'. As with most things in medicine, the goal posts are continually changing. We once used to say your blood pressure should be 100 plus your age. With this very loose definition, most people never made it to this level of blood pressure—or for that matter to the particular age that would give you that level of blood pressure. For example, if you're an 80-year-old and your blood pressure is around 180 systolic for too long, your body will soon know about it.

These days blood pressure is considered abnormal above 135/85 in people up to the age of 65 and above 140/90 in people beyond this age. A relatively recent article in the *New England Journal of Medicine*, however, has shown people with blood pressures in the high 'normal' range, defined as 130–140/80–90, still have around two-and-a-half times the rate of stroke and heart disease compared with people with a blood pressure in the normal range. Treatment aside, the lower your blood pressure, the better. If you can wander around with blood pressure of 90/60 without getting particularly dizzy, then this certainly serves your arteries well.

You may well ask, what is blood pressure anyway? Blood pressure is divided into two readings: the high reading, known as the systolic, and the low reading, known as the diastolic. That pulsating thing in your thorax known as your heart pumps blood around the body at a high pressure throughout the arteries. The blood then goes from the arteries to the arterioles, which are the pressure modulators in your tissues. From there the blood is delivered through the capillaries. After the oxygen and nutrients have been extracted at the capillary level, blood is delivered through the much lower-pressure venous system back to the right side of the heart, through the lungs, where it picks up oxygen, then back to the higher-pressure left side of the heart, where it starts pumping around the body yet again. A boring job, but someone's gotta do it!

The systolic pressure is related to the force of contraction of the heart. It is much more complex than this, but for the discussion of blood pressure, this description serves the argument well. As we age and everything begins to stiffen up (except for, of course, in the case of us males, certain areas tend to do the reverse), our major pipes become less elastic and, therefore, this contributes to the systolic pressure increasing.

The diastolic pressure, however, is related to what is happening in the arterioles, that is, the smaller blood vessels. This diastolic blood pressure is an indication of the resting tone in these arterioles.

The problem with having high blood pressure is that our bodies were only designed to cope with a particular pressure. Once we start rising above this pressure the tissues need protection so the arteries go into spasm. The rising blood pressure within the large to medium-size arteries then damages the lining of the blood vessels, allowing fat, cholesterol and white cells to infiltrate into the walls, setting up fatty plaques. The constant bombardment of blood vessels with high pressure can also weaken the walls themselves, contributing to cerebral haemorrhage (a bleed into the brain tissue) or another very serious condition known as aortic dissection. (Aortic dissection is an internal rupture of the main artery coming off the heart and, depending on the site of the dissection, unless treated immediately is often fatal.)

The common complications of high blood pressure are:

1. heart disease
2. stroke
3. renal disease
4. hypertensive eye changes.

Twenty to 30 years ago, before we had excellent treatment for high blood pressure, these complications were rife in the general public. Unfortunately, these days, it is still estimated that only around 50 per cent of cases of high blood pressure are diagnosed and of those, only 50 per cent have adequate treatment for their high blood pressure. Therefore, at any one time, only a quarter of the hypertensive population is receiving appropriate treatment.

As heart disease, stroke and kidney disease account for around 50 per cent of the deaths in our society, it is therefore vital to identify blood pressure early and to begin treatment as soon as possible.

Heart disease

High blood pressure is one of the major contributing risk factors to atherosclerotic coronary artery disease. High blood pressure also thickens the walls of the heart and is the most common cause of a condition known as congestive heart failure. The most common complication of high blood pressure is a rhythm disturbance in the heart known as atrial fibrillation.

The low-pressure chambers of the heart, known as the atria, continually pump blood into the high-pressure chambers, known as the ventricles. This is very hard work for these poor little atria and after a while they say, 'Forget it, fellas, I've had enough.' They 'quiver', and this quivering is the fibrillation. Then the ventricles lose their normal messages from the atria and beat all over the place. This chaotic rhythm can result in immediate reduction in cardiac output. The two major complications of developing atrial fibrillation are acute heart failure due to the disordered muscle contraction, and stroke.

When the atrium is quivering, the blood is not flushed through into the ventricles, therefore clots can form. If the heart then starts to contract normally, clots can be thrown off to the head causing a stroke. This is why, in people with either recurrent atrial fibrillation or atrial fibrillation that been present for greater than 48 hours, it is routine medical practice for the patient to be given a strong blood thinner, such as warfarin.

Stroke

This is a rather loose term meaning cerebrovascular disease—in other words, disease of the blood vessels going to the brain. Stroke usually means a thrombosis in one of the arteries but there are in fact many ways a stroke can manifest. The carotid arteries are the major blood supply to the front region of the brain. Carotid atherosclerosis (i.e. a build-up of fat in the carotid arteries) is a common cause of stroke. When a plaque in one of these arteries ruptures, it either obstructs the carotid arteries or, possibly, sends a shower of little clots further up into the cerebral circulation. Carotid atherosclerosis can be accurately and easily diagnosed with the use of a non-invasive technique known as carotid doppler. This employs ultrasound to visualise and measure the degree of obstruction in the carotid arteries. Atherosclerosis can, however, occur in the smaller blood vessels inside the brain and can also cause problems in the vertebral arteries at the back of the brain.

There is also another type of stroke, known as a Lacunar infarct, which affects the smaller blood vessels and usually improves over a few days or weeks. Often these types of strokes go relatively unnoticed, unlike the dramatic cerebral thrombosis that causes the sudden onset of weakness or paralysis down one side of the body and loss of speech. The heart (such as the case with atrial fibrillation) can also throw off small clots to the brain and this is called a cerebral embolus, yet another form of stroke. Finally, a cerebral haemorrhage, which is a bleed into the brain tissue, can cause sudden catastrophic problems and is part of the syndrome known as stroke.

Kidney disease

High blood pressure can affect the kidneys, the filter of the bloodstream. If the blood pressure is too high on a long-term basis, the kidneys develop thickening within the small arteries and then the filters, known as the glomerulus, become quite hardened and start to lose their function. High blood pressure–related kidney disease, however, has become quite rare in the modern era of more effective blood pressure treatment.

Causes of high blood pressure

If I line up 100 people with high blood pressure and investigate every organ in their body, looking for some particular abnormality, I will probably find abnormalities in between three and five people. Therefore, somewhere between 95 and 97 per cent have no obvious cause for their high blood pressure. The abnormalities that are found are known as secondary causes. The common secondary causes are as follows:

1. Chronic inflammation in the kidney, known as glomerulonephritis.
2. Obstruction to one of the arteries supplying the kidney, known as renal artery stenosis: This is either due to an abnormality in the blood-vessel wall known as fibro muscular dysplasia, which occurs in younger people, or atherosclerotic renal artery stenosis, which occurs more commonly in older people.
3. Other forms of chronic kidney disease.
4. Chronic kidney failure: Almost all people on renal dialysis have high blood pressure, especially just prior to dialysis. In people without normal kidneys they are very sensitive to shifts in fluid and any excessive fluid can push their blood pressure through the roof.
5. Problems with the adrenal gland: The adrenals are two little glands sitting on each of your kidneys, and are basically the stress glands in the body. The outer part of the adrenals, known as the adrenal cortex, makes the stress hormone cortisone and its related steroid hormones. The inner part of the adrenals, known as the adrenal medulla, makes the stress hormones adrenaline and noradrenaline. Very rarely, tumours can occur in either the cortex or the medulla, and these tumours can be associated with high blood pressure.
6. Aortic disease: A congenital obstruction in the aorta known as coarctation, it can also present as high blood pressure in young people.
7. Rare glandular disorders: Glandular disorders can be associated with high blood pressure, such as a tumour of the pituitary gland, a tumour of the parathyroid gland, etc.

Probably the most common association of high blood pressure, however, is the insulin resistance syndrome. The true mechanism of high blood pressure in insulin resistance is not as yet elucidated, but people who manifest the deadly quartet of tendency to diabetes, tendency to cholesterol abnormalities, tendency to obesity and tendency to hypertension commonly have hypertension as a central part of this syndrome.

So what about the 95 to 97 per cent of people with no obvious cause for their hypertension? These people have varying degrees of genetic metabolic abnormalities. Basically, metabolism is the way your cells perform their normal functions. If you had one of the common genetic aberrations setting you up for high blood pressure at some stage in your life and you lived in a more traditional society—spending your days gathering nuts and berries, fishing in the river and generally living without stress or pollution—then you would almost certainly not develop high blood pressure despite your genetically primed basal metabolism. You may die from total boredom, but you certainly wouldn't die from a complication of high blood pressure. In our society, however, your blood pressure would rise. Sure, if you are the sort of person I described in the first paragraph of this section—the ranting, raving, 'throw-things-at-people' type—you will probably develop your high blood pressure much earlier than the more laid-back among us.

SALT
High blood pressure usually manifests itself after the age of 40, although I have seen many people with high blood pressure before this age. With the constant bombardment of our bodies with salt up to this point, the metabolism finally caves in and thus, high blood pressure results. If, however, you have developed high blood pressure, you only have a 30 per cent chance of being able to reduce your blood pressure by salt restriction.

I don't know how many times I am told by different patients that they don't eat salt so, therefore, why do they have high blood pressure? The reality is that our bodies probably only need somewhere between 40 and 80 milliequivalents of salt per day to survive. An average, low-salt

Western diet takes in somewhere between 120 and 150 milliequivalents of salt a day, and many people are pushing that up to the 200–300-milliequivalent range. They have been bombarding their bodies with this amount of salt for so long that their metabolic systems have re-adjusted and pushed their blood pressure higher. Even if they then markedly restrict their salt, they will not always return their blood pressure to normal.

It is also not just the salt causing the problem. It is the interaction between sodium, potassium, magnesium, calcium and water. All of these substances are vital constituents of cell metabolism and are all involved in the messages transmitted between the nerves, the blood vessels and other cells. If our cells contain excessive sodium due to a combination of defective metabolism and constant bombardment with dietary salt, eventually the cells become salty and waterlogged and do not relax properly. Combine this with a dietary deficiency of potassium, calcium and magnesium and you're well on your way to starting your high blood pressure career.

FIVE-DAY SALT TEST

If you really love your salt and are thinking, 'If I keep doing this I'm going to put my blood pressure through the roof at some stage in my life', why not try my five-day salt test.

Rent or buy a home blood pressure–monitoring kit. Check your blood pressure a few times a day for a week or so, to establish a normal pattern to your blood pressure. During this time, continue with your normal diet. Once you have established a pattern to your blood pressure, follow a very rigid salt restriction:

1. No salt on the table.
2. No salt in the cooking.
3. Avoid obvious salty foods, including all takeaway food, any processed or packaged foods laden with salt, products such as commercial peanut butter, Vegemite, tomato sauce, margarine, cheese, organ meats and mineral water.

During the period of salt restriction closely monitor your blood pressure three to four times per day. If your blood pressure has registered a drop greater than 5 in both systolic and/or diastolic pressure, then you probably have a degree of salt sensitivity and would benefit from ongoing salt restriction.

You can perform this test whether you do or don't have current high blood pressure.

It is my feeling that salt should be restricted if you suffer from one of the following complaints:

1. established high blood pressure
2. strong family history of high blood pressure
3. heart disease
4. kidney disease or other states of fluid retention
5. abnormal results from the five-day salt test.

Case study: Vanessa Schmidt—Vanessa Schmidt is a 43-year-old woman with long-standing high blood pressure. She consulted me as she was keen on reducing her current medication. Vanessa had reasonable control of her blood pressure but this was by no means perfect. I had put her on a combined A-2 inhibitor and diuretic and was still achieving blood pressure levels of only 145/95–100.

She then admitted to me that she very much enjoyed salt and really couldn't live without adding it to most foods. I asked her to follow my five-day salt plan and she found her blood pressure dropped to a low–normal range purely because of the marked restriction in her salt intake. In Vanessa's case, she was obviously salt-sensitive and restricting salt was the major intervention that would help prevent ongoing problems.

Professor Michael Alderman from the Albert Einstein College of Medicine in New York does not agree that everyone should be restricting salt. Back in 1997 his research team began analysing the diets of

11 000 people. In 1998, they published the results in *The Lancet*, suggesting that recommendations to lower salt across the board may be harmful. Professor Alderman's team found death rates were inversely related to salt intake. Strangely enough, the more salt people ingested, the less likely they were to die from cardiovascular disease. To understand how this somewhat paradoxic conclusion can possibly have some scientific basis, you have to understand how this magical thing called 'our body' works.

Within the body are a whole series of control systems and feedback loops maintaining homeostasis, that is, the normal balance of our day-to-day metabolism. The body is designed to be able to cope with large shifts in fluid. There are times when we ingest far too much in the way of salt and water, and there are other times when we become dehydrated. Because of this, 'the Great Designer' threw in all these extra chemicals allowing us to cope with these extremes. One of the wonderful fluid balance systems is known as the renin-angiotensin system.

When there is any drop in the blood pressure or drop in fluid going through the kidneys, a chemical known as renin is released, which eventually switches on the production of a substance known as angiotensin-2. Angiotensin-2 is the most powerful vaso-constrictor (blood vessel constrictor) in the body. When your fluid is down or your blood pressure is low, the angiotensin-2 constricts the blood vessels, attempting to restore your blood pressure back to normal. Angiotensin-2 also releases another hormone known as aldosterone, which forces the kidney to retain salt and water, thus also assisting in maintaining your blood pressure even further.

If you are not one of these people plagued by high blood pressure or a strong family history of high blood pressure, using a bit of salt suppresses the release of renin and therefore reduces the amount of angiotensin-2 produced. Too much angiotensin-2 is not good for the heart because the constriction can help contribute to the rupturing of plaques in the heart, or also in the carotid arteries. If you do not fit into the aforementioned categories, I believe having a moderate amount of salt may even be of some benefit.

Salt is not the only metabolic aberration leading to high blood pressure. Many people with high blood pressure are born with an abnormal gene generating too much of this angiotensin-2 stuff in their bloodstream, therefore constricting the blood vessels and eventually putting up their blood pressure. As I will discuss later, we now have wonderful agents that directly block this angiotensin-2, and are useful agents in the management of high blood pressure.

Diagnosing high blood pressure

To establish a diagnosis of high blood pressure, it is important not to take one isolated reading. Multiple readings at different times of the day are a much better and more accurate method. If somebody has just rushed in late for their appointment after a rather intense business meeting and their blood pressure is too high, I would basically ignore this level. I would, however, suggest that this person has their blood pressure checked on a few more occasions. Personally, I am more interested in blood pressure readings taken by a person at home or at work than I would be when they come to visit me. Often a visit to the doctor means anxiety on the part of the patient or, at times, sitting in a waiting room relaxing for half an hour to an hour before they can get in to see the doctor, so I'm not particularly impressed with the accuracy of these blood pressure readings.

Many studies have shown that 24-hour blood pressure monitoring allows a much more accurate assessment of high blood pressure than do isolated office visits. I am a big supporter of the concept of self-monitoring. Sensible self-monitoring is an extremely accurate way to determine true blood pressure readings so long as there is close correlation between your doctor's machine and your machine. The readings you obtain at home and at work are of much more use to the doctor than their own readings. The newer home monitoring devices are very accurate. I would, however, like to bring in a word of caution. Unfortunately, I have seen far too many patients who have developed an obsession with their health. The more home monitoring devices they have, the more time they spend monitoring themselves.

HOME MONITORING

Often, home monitoring becomes so excessive that I have seen quite a number of people arrive at my office with pages of blood pressure readings, weight charts, fluid balance charts and notes on every manner of minor symptoms and complaints they have had over the preceding few months. Some people file their pathology results in chronological order and keep a constant record of every medical visit they have had. Although, at times, this is useful for the doctor, I believe it is counter-productive for almost all patients. Interestingly, it is my observation that almost all people who do this are not particularly ill in the first place. One could argue that this obsessive self-monitoring prevents them from being ill, but I believe it prevents the 'stopping and smelling the roses' concept to some extent. This is sadly lacking in our society. I saw a couple a few weeks ago in my practice where the wife had her blood pressure measured 10 times in one day and on each occasion the blood pressure was normal. I feel it is important to achieve a middle path when embarking on a self-monitoring program. By all means, monitor your health, but don't become obsessed with it.

To establish a diagnosis of high blood pressure you need at least three, and preferably six, readings on different occasions above 135/85. If you are over the age of 65, raise this to greater than 140/90. If you are diabetic or have the insulin resistance syndrome, any pressure above 130/80 should be considered abnormal, therefore, treatment should be commenced at a much earlier phase.

WHEN SHOULD PEOPLE BE INVESTIGATED FOR SECONDARY CAUSES?

William Funnell is a 48-year-old, stressed executive whose father died at the age of 52 of a cerebral haemorrhage. William's father had high blood pressure for 10 years and William has a blood pressure of 160/110 with a pulse rate of 96 per minute. He weighs 100 kilograms and is 175 centimetres tall.

It would be highly unlikely that William had a secondary cause for high blood pressure in these circumstances. Before I commence treatment, however, I would perform a simple inexpensive screen, such as a urinalysis, looking for protein and blood, fasting blood tests including cholesterol, triglyceride, HDL, blood sugar level, uric acid and urea, electrolytes, and creatinine (assessment of kidney function). Optional testing in this setting would be either CT scanning of the coronary arteries and/or a stress echocardiogram. The stress echocardiogram measures the thickness of the walls of the heart, which is a very important prognostic feature of high blood pressure. This is known as left ventricular hypertrophy and it is a major predictor for heart attack and stroke. The stress component is important, firstly to diagnose any silent lack of oxygen to the heart muscle, and also to determine its response to blood pressure during exertion. When William performed an exercise test his blood pressure rose to 230/120. A blood pressure rising above 200/100 during exertion is a very poor prognostic feature of high blood pressure. This suggests William should have very aggressive treatment for his blood pressure. The CT scan would give an indication of how much atherosclerosis was or wasn't present in Bill's arteries as a consequence of his lifestyle and high blood pressure.

If I assessed a 25-year-old female with no family history of high blood pressure but is found on a routine screen for a job application to have a blood pressure of 180/120, I would then look for a secondary cause for her condition. The problem in this setting is she would still only have a 10 per cent chance of having a condition, such as fibromuscular dysplasia of her renal arteries, glomerulonephritis, etc., but it is still more important to search for this cause.

Non-drug therapy

If your initial assessment shows that there has already been quite significant organ problems, or a marked hypertensive response to exercise, or very high 24-hour blood pressure control, then I believe it is important to start drug therapy rather quickly. If, however, your blood pressures are in the mid to moderate range, you have significant room to move with lifestyle modification. If there is no evidence of left ventricular hypertrophy with a reasonable blood pressure response to exercise, then you could probably start on six months of lifestyle modification and have your blood pressure re-evaluated frequently during this time. The five-step natural approach to reducing blood pressure is:

1. dietary intervention
2. weight loss
3. regular physical exercise
4. alcohol restriction
5. behavioural techniques.

1. DIETARY INTERVENTION

I have already mentioned the importance of salt restriction, especially in people who are salt-sensitive. Increasing the calcium, magnesium and potassium content of your diet can also help in reducing your blood pressure. Recent studies of dietary intervention have shown a significant benefit. Even the simple habit of increasing your fruit and vegetable intake to the suggested two or three pieces of fruit and three to five servings of vegetables per day can cause a significant reduction in blood pressure.

Because nuts contain a wonderful chemical called L-arginine, ingesting 10 to 15 nuts a day may also assist in dropping blood pressure. Nuts are also a rich source of minerals, in particular, magnesium and potassium. Low-fat dairy food is also of significant value in reducing blood pressure. Interestingly, in a recent study that monitored a group of people aged between 18 and 30 for many years, the rates of the insulin resistance syndrome, of which high blood pressure is a prominent feature, were found to be much lower in those that had the highest dairy consumption.

2. WEIGHT LOSS
A significant loss of weight can also lead to a significant reduction in blood pressure.

3. REGULAR PHYSICAL EXERCISE
There is no doubt there is an interplay between exercise and weight loss, but exercise itself, regardless of weight loss, can help to lower blood pressure. The suggested regimen is in the section on exercise later in this book.

4. ALCOHOL RESTRICTION
Although I support the use of low-dose alcohol consumption, there is no doubt that extending your consumption beyond the standard one to two drinks per day will directly increase your blood pressure.

> **Case study: Robert Wright**—Robert Wright is 41 years old. He came to me for management of high blood pressure. On further questioning, Robert had great difficulty sleeping. In fact, he was consuming six or seven small bottles of beer (the equivalent of 15 grams of alcohol per bottle), which he stated was the only way he could sleep at night. His wife complained to me that he was a very heavy snorer and that he would wake at two or three in the morning after a few hours' sleep and find it almost impossible to resume his slumber.
>
> When I convinced Robert to cut back his drinking to two small glasses of alcohol per day, his sleeping patterns improved and his blood pressure returned to normal.

There is a misconception on the part of many people that alcohol helps sleep. What alcohol does is acutely act as a sedative which can precipitate a disordered form of sleep. Normal sleeping patterns are affected by alcohol.

One of the most common reasons for disrupted sleep, especially for males, is sleep apnoea. This is known as the snorers' disease. We basically sleep so we can have a few cycles of deep sleep during the night.

These cycles last for around 30 minutes and usually occur on four to five occasions. During this cycle of sleep, which is non-dreaming deep sleep, we rejuvenate our body's systems. If you suffer sleep apnoea, the muscles in the back of the throat become very lax. When you drift into a deep sleep the airway starts to close over and you begin snoring. When you reach the stage of very deep sleep and your muscles are totally relaxed, the throat totally closes and the airway blocks. Your body then has to make the decision as to whether you stay in deep sleep without breathing (which is a little state called death) or return to a light phase of sleeping. The next day you will feel dog-tired.

Consuming excessive amounts of alcohol is a very good way of worsening sleep apnoea. Having these recurrent bursts of lack of oxygen and apnoeic spells throughout the night also precipitates a rise in blood pressure.

Not everyone consuming more than two glasses of alcohol will push up their blood pressure through these means, but this is a very good way to develop established high blood pressure if you combine too much alcohol with sleep apnoea.

5. BEHAVIOURAL TECHNIQUES

Behavioural techniques, such as biofeedback, meditation or relaxation therapy, have been shown to reduce blood pressure by significant levels. In his book *Perfect Blood Pressure Naturally*, Dr David Lovell-Smith clearly demonstrates the extraordinary effect of transcendental meditation in the lowering of blood pressure. Dr Lovell-Smith presents well over 100 scientific references in support of his argument, and for those of you experiencing problems with blood pressure who would prefer not to start on lifelong medication, I suggest you either purchase his book or contact a meditation teacher and start the practice immediately. Not only would you experience the enormous health benefits of meditation, but it is a wonderful introduction to a more enriching, peaceful life.

Case study: Kelvin Jones—Just the other day, I saw Kelvin Jones. Kelvin is 48 years old and works as a bricklayer. He has not been especially diligent with his lifestyle. Although he is not a particularly heavy drinker, he does have abdominal obesity, a slight elevation in his blood sugar and is not careful with his diet. He has tried numerous blood pressure treatments, all of which have caused some variety of side effect.

Kelvin wanted to know why he had high blood pressure and what else could be done, apart from taking drugs, to help him lower his blood pressure. He had already had extensive investigations and all the secondary causes for high blood pressure were excluded. When I discussed non-pharmacologic therapy, he suggested he'd already tried these different methods and none of them had worked. He was a self-confessed highly stressed person and did admit that when he took an anti-anxiety medication, his blood pressure dropped.

When I suggested meditation, he thought I was some type of wierdo. Basically, Kelvin had come to me for some sort of magic that does not exist. The best way to manage blood pressure after you have excluded the secondary causes is to bring in as many lifestyle techniques as possible; but then, if your blood pressure is still above the designated levels, you need drug therapy.

Pharmalogical therapies

There is no doubt that if you put an enormous effort into the non-pharmacologic side of blood pressure management you will obtain a significant drop in your blood pressure. Unfortunately, many people subconsciously prefer the push-button answer of swallowing a pill every day, although they give great lip service to the fact that they really don't want to take a pill for the rest of their life.

When the pharmaceutical world was in its infancy, the drugs available had all manner of side effects from depression to impotence, and/or a combination of both. Today's drugs are not without their side effects and it is unfortunate that probably around 5 to 10 per cent of people who take any medication will develop some type of reaction to the drug. These reactions are usually not of a serious nature, but are certainly enough to affect the quality of someone's life. If you have to swallow a pill for the rest of your life, you certainly will not—and should not—accept a significant side effect.

One of the other problems with using blood pressure drugs is if you take 100 people with the same level of blood pressure and treat them with the same drug, only around 50 or 60 will achieve normal blood pressure levels with that one agent. An additional 30 to 40 people will require two agents, and the last 10 to 20 may need multiple drugs to achieve normal blood pressure control. There is absolutely no way of predicting which people will suffer side effects and who will respond well to treatment.

There are five main groups of drugs used, with many other drugs on the drawing board and quite a number of reasonable back-up drugs if one of the five causes a problem. I must make a point very strongly, however: *if you have been well controlled on an older-style drug for many years without any problems, there is absolutely no point in changing.* Your body has not become accustomed to the drugs so they do not lose their affect, nor if you have been taking them for 20 to 30 years will there be some nasty problem lurking in the background.

I well remember the case of a man in his seventies who was extremely well controlled on a cocktail of very old drugs that usually cause horrendous side effects in most people. This man had no side effects and was progressing well with normal blood pressure control. When his doctor went on holiday a new locum took over and was horrified by the combination this man was swallowing. He immediately said, 'We have something so much better than these treatments.' The patient started on a new batch of blood pressure treatments and within three weeks he was on a kidney machine, fighting for his life. A few weeks later he suffered a stroke and died a month after this.

I am not in any way suggesting these new drugs are dangerous and should be avoided. In this man's case he had a very rare reaction to one of the new drugs and was not monitored correctly. So, the point I am making from this is that if you're on a regimen that is working for you, don't change.

The five main groups of drugs for blood pressure treatment are:

1. diuretics
2. beta blockers
3. ACE inhibitors
4. angiotensin-2 inhibitors
5. calcium antagonists.

Blood pressure tends to be the end result of many different metabolic abnormalities. In a younger person (less than 55), the major underlying abnormality tends to be a switching on of the sympathetic (fear–fight–flight) system. The best initial drugs to treat this type of blood pressure is either the ACE inhibitors, the A-2 inhibitors or the beta blockers. In people over the age of 55 with high blood pressure, this tends to be more related to a stiffening of the pipes, so treatment with diuretics or the calcium antagonists tends to be more appropriate. I must state, however, that this is purely a guideline and not a hard and fast rule.

The other groups occasionally used are the centrally acting drugs, other vaso-dilating drugs and the other forms of neuronal or nerve blockers. Before you embark on blood pressure treatment it is important to note the following points:

- There is no 'one-pill-fits-all' treatment. Just because your next-door neighbour responded beautifully to a blood pressure drug, it does not mean you will. It may take a trial of a number of pills before you find the one suitable for you.
- In my opinion it is better to be on two or three pills at a low dose than it is to continually increase the dose of one drug. The higher the dose of one drug, the more potential for side effects. The other advantage of using a combination medication is the ability to treat blood pressure from a few different metabolic angles. We now have an increasing number of preparations where two different blood pressure medications are combined in the one pill, making compliance so much easier.
- It is a much better principle to take a pill once a day than to have to take a pill two to three times a day. Usually the once-a-day pills have a much longer action, therefore they achieve much smoother blood pressure control.

NIGHT OR DAY?

I am always somewhat amused when I hear of people taking their blood pressure pills at night. The reasoning for this is that strokes occur more commonly in the early hours of the morning and you are therefore covering this period by taking a blood pressure pill before you go to bed. This is very foolish thinking. Strokes related to high blood pressure occur because of poor blood pressure control throughout the 24-hour period. Your blood pressure is almost always at its highest during the day, falling slightly during the evening and at its lowest while you're asleep. If you take a blood pressure pill prior to sleep, your blood pressure will fall even further, thus creating a marked discrepancy between your waking blood pressure and your sleeping blood pressure. Often it is this marked difference in pressure that can lead to a stroke. I am not saying I never prescribe blood pressure pills for night-time use, but I always prefer my patients to take all their blood pressure medications first thing in the morning.

- There is a strong temptation to start treatment and then assume your blood pressure does not require constant monitoring. Only around 25 per cent of those with high blood pressure have adequate control at any time. It is vital to aim for target blood pressure levels and achieve these levels whether it takes multiple medications or not. There are significant consequences of poor blood pressure control and great benefits for having normal blood pressure.
- In almost all cases, blood pressure treatment is lifelong. One of the problems with any chronic illness is drug compliance. Unfortunately, around 50 per cent of people have stopped taking their medications 12 months after the initial prescription and the medications only work for the time you are swallowing them. With such a large selection of newer drugs with fewer side effects, there is almost always a medication or combination of treatments that can lead to excellent blood pressure control.

High blood pressure is a major risk for heart disease and many other complications within the vascular system. It is vital to recognise elevations in blood pressure early on and to have them effectively managed. The only way to know you have a problem with your blood pressure is to have your blood pressure checked. Every time you visit a doctor once you are over the age of 35, he should routinely check your blood pressure whether you have attended for a sore throat, a pain in your ankle or even for a flu vaccination. Having your blood pressure checked is the most inexpensive, effective form of cardiovascular screening that has ever been invented.

OTHER RISK FACTORS

I have devoted a significant amount of space to the discussion of cholesterol, to put it into perspective. Although I believe it is important to treat high cholesterol, I certainly do not believe that an isolated high reading is the cause of heart disease, nor do I believe it is the major reason we develop atherosclerosis. There are numerous risk factors operative in the generation of atherosclerosis, I will continue the discussion of these in the remainder of this chapter.

Diabetes

There is a misconception regarding diabetes: you either have it or you don't. Although in basic terms this is obviously true, having the predisposition to diabetes (i.e. being insulin-resistant) is not as bad but it still requires early detection and management. In reality, diabetes is part of the continuum of insulin resistance. If you are insulin-resistant but not as yet diabetic, it means that your pancreas is still producing enough insulin to maintain a normal blood sugar level. By the time you have had a firm diagnosis of diabetes made, your pancreas cannot keep up the production of insulin for your body's needs and, therefore, starts to fail.

Another interesting misconception is insulin-dependent versus non-insulin-dependent diabetes. In most cases, insulin-dependent diabetes is a condition presenting in childhood, characterised by relatively sudden loss of pancreatic function. The pancreas is damaged by, presumably, a viral attack (or possibly some other toxin) in a genetically predisposed person, leading to the cessation of production of insulin by the pancreas. Without immediate and lifelong insulin therapy, the person develops a condition known as diabetic ketoacidosis, which eventually leads to a coma and death.

Some very creative laboratories around the world are developing pancreatic transplant techniques and islet cell (the cells that make insulin) transplant techniques, and other laboratories have even used immune suppression therapy in an attempt to restore pancreatic function. Without ongoing monitoring and exquisite control of blood sugar, these young insulin-dependent diabetic sufferers commonly progress to premature cardiovascular disease, renal disease where their kidneys fail, loss of function of the peripheral nerves and severe eye problems—depending on the degree of control of the diabetes. This process may take 20 to 30 years after the diagnosis, even less for some people, while others are much luckier and can cope with this condition without major complications.

Insulin-dependent diabetes, however, only accounts for around 5 to 10 per cent of the entire diabetic population. The much more common type of diabetes is non-insulin-dependent diabetes, which occurs usually over the age of 40 and is often associated with the other features of the insulin resistant syndrome: high blood pressure, cholesterol abnormalities and obesity.

Although there is a distinct genetic abnormality for insulin resistance, lifestyle factors play a very important role. Not infrequently, these people will develop such severe pancreatic failure that they will require insulin. They are still not insulin-*dependent*, only insulin-*requiring*. The distinction here is, if you stop insulin therapy in these people, they will not develop ketoacidosis because they still have enough residual pancreatic function to prevent this deadly condition. Their blood sugar will, however, rise to dangerous levels and will require treatment.

Even in people with insulin resistance, the risk for cardiovascular disease is markedly elevated. Once diabetes occurs the rates of heart disease and stroke go through the roof. Again, in most cases, this is entirely preventable with aggressive lifestyle modification and appropriate medical therapy. As with all conditions, the diabetic who puts more effort into swallowing their pills than losing weight through sensible eating and sensible exercise is following a very foolish path. Diabetic medications are a bandaid without lifestyle modification. The bandaid itself is not performing any healing function, only masking the underlying consequences of the disease.

Lipoprotein(a)

When I am speaking to a professional group or at a large corporate convention, I often ask the question, 'Who in the audience has heard of lipoprotein(a)?' In a group of 300 to 400 people I would be lucky to have one or two hands go up (usually because these people had read my books previously). In fact, one in five people in Western society have an elevated level of lipoprotein(a) in their bloodstream.

Lipoprotein(a) is a vicious cause of premature vascular disease. Most of the prospective studies performed on it have shown a 70 per cent increase in risk for vascular disease in those people whose levels are above 0.3 millimoles per litre. Lipoprotein(a) (Lp(a)) is a large molecule travelling around the bloodstream with an LDL molecule in its head and a large apoprotein(a) molecule dangling behind. The LDL is easily oxidised and promotes the build-up of fat in the arterial wall. This is regardless of the total cholesterol levels, although the combination of a high cholesterol and a high Lp(a) can promote vicious heart disease if not treated. The apoprotein(a) part of the molecule has a tendency to thicken the blood, therefore, Lp(a) performs undesirable actions, such as:

(i)   promote fat build-up in the wall of arteries
(ii) thickens the blood.

Mainstream science as yet does not have any good answers as to why we have Lp(a). For a reasonable explanation we must revisit Linus Pauling, the Vitamin C man. He was considered by mainstream medicine as a zealot and something of a lunatic. This lunatic, however, was the father of molecular biology and also won two unshared Nobel prizes (the only person in the history of the world to do so). He died in his mid-nineties still working 10 to 12 hours a day.

I must say from the outset that I believe it is important to have a healthy suspicion of any theory that tries to encompass one explanation for most of the world's ills. Many of Pauling's theories were based around the observation that human beings cannot produce their own Vitamin C. Most animals *can* produce their own Vitamin C and don't appear to develop atherosclerosis. Most animals, however, do not consume the highly processed synthetic diets we do, and once you introduce these foods into many of these so-called Vitamin C–producing animals, they will very rapidly develop atherosclerosis.

I still believe there is some credence to his theories, and I have seen in many cases a dramatic response to therapy that uses a combination of Vitamin C and lysine for patients with a high Lp(a).

The Pauling–Rath Hypothesis

Vitamin C is an essential chemical for many normal bodily functions. One of the main actions of Vitamin C is in the formation of collagen. Collagen is the major supporting protein in the body, being a normal part of blood vessels, the skin and other supporting structures. Without Vitamin C, these supporting structures break down very easily and if you withdraw a healthy supply of Vitamin C from anyone's diet, they will soon develop scurvy.

We need a plentiful daily supply of Vitamin C and the B group for normal body metabolism. If we have bouts of Vitamin C lack (i.e. bouts of scurvy), our blood vessels become weak and break down. The Pauling–Rath Hypothesis states that Lp(a) evolved as an attempted antidote to scurvy. The clinical manifestation of scurvy is the breaking down of blood-vessels and bleeding into the gums and other tissues, such as muscles. Lp(a) puts some fat into the blood-vessel wall in people who are malnourished and therefore lack fat. It also thickens the blood around a broken, weakened blood vessel, therefore plugging the hole. And so, Vitamin C in high doses acts as an antidote to Lp(a).

Pauling also suggests the use of L-lysine and L-proline, two amino acids that coat the Lp(a) molecule and prevent it from hooking into the blood-vessel wall. He states that at least 3 grams of Vitamin C, L-lysine and L-proline should be used, but in my experience, I have had success with lower doses. Routinely, I use 2 grams of Vitamin C along with 500mg of L-lysine daily.

If you screen a group of people who have suffered some form of vascular disease—heart attack, stroke or peripheral vascular disease—before the age of 55, somewhere between 30 and 40 per cent of them will have elevated levels of Lp(a) in their bloodstream. I believe the management of Lp(a) is multi-factorial.

DIET
Although Lp(a) is a strongly genetic factor, there has been a few studies to show higher levels of Lp(a) associated with the consumption of excessive trans fatty acids. There is also some work to show a significant reduction in Lp(a) levels with fish consumption.

MANAGING CHOLESTEROL
If I have patients with a high calcium score on the CT scanner and an elevated Lp(a), I tend to aggressively manage their cholesterol regardless of their total cholesterol levels. This, of course, flies in the face of all the recommended government guidelines, but I am treating human beings, not medical statistics. The only time I would not bother managing cholesterols in this setting is if the total cholesterol level was less than 4.

NICOTINIC ACID (NIACIN/VITAMIN B3)
If I suffered significant vascular disease or had a calcium score well above 400, unless my cholesterol was below 4, I would take a combination of a statin and nicotinic acid—regardless. If there is evidence of a high calcium and your Lp(a) is elevated, you should certainly consider this approach. How much nicotinic acid is necessary to lower Lp(a)? The answer to this is: the more, the better. At least 1 gram a day is important and preferably, the immediate-acting stuff if you can tolerate the flushing. I have had some patients being able to consume up to 3 grams a day. In the United States, where they have better slow-release preparations, patients are taking up to 7 grams a day. Even with doses of 1 gram a day

you can hope to reduce Lp(a) by around 30 per cent. I have had some patients follow my entire regimen and bring their Lp(a) back to normal.

VITAMIN THERAPY

Again, as always, it's your body—not mine. If it were me, I would strongly advise the combination of Vitamin C and L-lysine. You, however, may be on either side of the fence. If you are a more conservative person, the medical evidence *strongly* supports the combination of a statin and nicotinic acid to markedly reduce your risk for further vascular events. If you are more a Linus Pauling devotee, you may even be prepared to take high doses of Vitamin C along with L-lysine and proline. For those of you interested in more information, there is an excellent website. Using the search engine on your computer, type in: lipoprotein(a) linked in with Linus Pauling. There are well over 20 pages of excellent information.

HORMONE REPLACEMENT THERAPY

There was a recent trial known as the HERS study, looking at hormone replacement therapy in women with vascular disease. In fact, the only women who derived a significant benefit from hormone replacement therapy were those women with an elevated level of Lp(a). Hormone replacement therapy reduces Lp(a) levels and, thus, one of the major reasons hormone replacement therapy causes benefit in women with vascular disease.

Whether male hormone replacement therapy with testosterone has a similar effect is yet to be proven. It is interesting that around 50 per cent of males over the age of 45 do go through a similar loss of hormonal function, which has the interesting name of andropause. The features of andropause are loss of erectile function, lack of libido, fatigue, aches and pains, and irritability. Most males would never admit to any of these symptoms, but I am sure there are many females reading this section who will agree I have just described their partner. There are many proponents of male hormone replacement therapy but it is important to stress (just as a female should have regular checks for breast cancer with self-examintion, a medical assessment and mammography) that men should have regular checks for prostate cancer with a PSA, digital rectal examination and possibly prostatic ultrasound—especially prior to commencing therapy with male hormone replacement. Also, in the same way that women have assessments of their hormonal levels, men can also have testosterone and DHEA levels measured.

I have stated that having a high level of Lp(a) in your bloodstream increases your risk for vascular disease by about 70 per cent. It is interesting that around 30 per cent of people with high levels do not suffer any vascular disease. One of the explanations for this is that there are varying types of Lp(a). In fact, I have screened many patients with extremely high levels of Lp(a) and it is my feeling that those with the very high levels tend to have less vascular disease than those with Lp(a) levels in the intermediate range—from 0.3 up to 1.5. As yet, I have not performed a formal study and this is certainly only an impression from having screened over 15 000 patients with Lp(a) and CT screening. My hypothesis (not as yet scientifically confirmed) is that very high levels of Lp(a) have larger Lp(a) structures and find it harder to traverse the blood-vessel wall, therefore, they have less propensity to cause fatty plaques. This may be a load of cobblers, but it certainly requires further research.

Homocysteine

Elevated levels of homocysteine in the bloodstream occur in around 10 per cent of any community and about 30 to 40 per cent of people with premature vascular disease. Homocysteine is basically a toxic by-product of methionine, which is one of the essential amino acids present in all protein sources containing the nine essential amino acids.

Around 10 per cent of the community has a minor gene defect which allows any excess methionine to be shunted towards homocysteine. The problem with homocysteine is its ability to erode the lining of blood vessels, therefore causing endothelial dysfunction, and also to thicken the blood by making those sticky cells, known as platelets, aggregate together.

Most of the prospective work on homocysteine has shown if your levels are above 10 micromoles per litre, your risk for vascular disease is well over three times the normal level. Most of the people with minor elevations in homocysteine over this level have a common genetic abnormality of an enzyme known as 5, 10 methyltetrahydrofolate reductase. The other sufferers of a high homocysteine have more significant problems. The first defect requires therapy with folic acid and B12, whereas the second defect is more B6-dependent.

I have had a few patients who are refractory to treatment with vitamins and this is almost always because they have either a severe medical problem such as kidney disease, or more commonly have a B12 deficiency—usually caused by pernicious anaemia.

The most rewarding aspect of finding an elevated homocysteine is the ease of treatment. The simple addition of a good-quality, natural multi-vitamin with 400 micrograms of folic acid can restore homocysteine levels back to normal in most cases. There are, as yet, no long-term studies to show that vitamin therapy in the treatment of a high homocysteine will arrest, reverse or prevent vascular disease. But the weight of evidence is so strong, I do not hesitate to use the suggested multi-vitamin combination in these cases.

Highly sensitive C-reactive protein (hs-CRP)

C-reactive protein is known as an acute-phase reactant. Basically, this means any inflammatory or infective process in the body that stimulates the production of a number of proteins and other chemicals. Many of these proteins are purely markers for this inflammatory or infective process.

Many years ago, my eldest daughter developed Rubella at the age of 18 months. Unfortunatey, I caught it from her as an episode of moderate Rubella encephalitis. At the time I was working as a registrar in one of Sydney's kidney units, and I could not attend work. When we were working at the renal unit we had to give blood as a control measure. When I gave blood a couple of weeks after this episode of Rubella encephalitis, my immune complexes (one of the acute-phase reactants) were 66 per cent—the normal range for the laboratory at that stage was less than 20 per cent. This was two weeks after I had recovered. I could just imagine the amount of proteins that were running around my bloodstream.

C-reactive protein is probably the most common acute-phase reactant and has been shown in recent work to also cause some damage of its own, and not just to be elevated as a consequence of inflammation. If there is an obvious reason for the rise in C-reactive protein, such as arthritis or an acute infection, this is not as concerning from a cardiac viewpoint as the person who has a long-standing elevation of C-reactive protein. If this occurs without any obvious cause for the inflammation, it suggests that the possessor of the elevated C-reactive protein has a more switched-on immune system than someone who is in the lower range for this protein. You would think that this means they have a stronger immune system, but in fact, it means their white cells are probably more reactive and, therefore, in the case of cardiac disease, the white cells can eat away at a fatty plaque causing the plaque to rupture.

A recent review of C-reactive protein revealed that levels in the higher range were slightly more predictive for acute vascular events, such as sudden death and heart attack, than were cholesterol levels. If someone has an elevated cholesterol and a high C-reactive protein they have a huge increase in vascular events. At this stage, C-reactive protein, especially in its newest and most accurate form (highly sensitive C-reactive protein), is not being measured routinely as a risk marker for heart disease. We hear the usual catch-cry, 'More research is needed before any suggestions can be made.' This is despite the fact that numerous studies have now confirmed the link between an elevated level of C-reactive protein and risk for heart disease.

INFECTION AND INFLAMMATION

An elevated level of highly sensitive C-reactive protein may be present purely because of a combination of genetic and metabolic factors, predisposing a person to have a more sensitive inflammatory system. It therefore promotes the build-up of fat in your arteries and the subsequent rupturing of these fatty plaques. In a number of cases, however, there are more specific causes for the switching on of your immune system, such as a chronic inflammatory state or an acute or chronic infective process. There are many suggested culprits for this switching on of the inflammatory system, the most common being one of three infections:

1. Chlamydia Pneumoniae: This is a common infection, often causing a non-specific pneumonia. Significant research points to Chlamydia Pneumonia being present in many atherosclerotic plaques. If you examine the blood of people with heart disease, only a proportion will have evidence of a prior infection with Chlamydia Pneumonia. If you remove some of the fatty plaque (via a catheter during an angiogram), almost all the plaque will contain evidence of chlamydial infection. The question here is: is the infection a cause for promoting atherosclerosis or does it just like hanging around in fatty plaques to have a bit of a feast? No-one really knows the answer, but there have been a handful of studies where people were treated with specific antibiotics to kill bugs, such as Chlamydia, and some have shown a significant reduction in further cardiac events in those treated.
2. Helicobacter Pylori: Helicobacter Pylori is the major cause of peptic ulceration. When a Perth researcher, Professor Barry Marshall, suggested the link between Helicobacter infection and peptic ulceration, he was ridiculed at the time. Some researchers have since found high levels of Helicobacter titres in people with heart disease.
3. Cytomegalovirus: The common virus has also been found in higher levels in people with heart disease.

I am not suggesting that atherosclerosis, heart attacks, and all the other sequelae are caused by infections, but there is no doubt that the three bugs I have just mentioned, and possibly numerous other bugs, may in some way contribute to the acceleration or progression of heart disease. Therefore, using appropriate antibiotic therapy as part of the treatment may be the way of the future.

Thrombotic (pro-clotting) states

Atherosclerosis (the progressive build-up of fat, calcium and other scar tissue in the arteries) is a very slow process—it may take decades for a person to have evidence of substantial atherosclerosis. The entire process confines itself to the wall of the artery, in most cases, and may never progress to become a blockage of the channel itself.

Heart attack, sudden death or severe angina are not caused by athero-sclerosis per se, but by the rupture through the wall into the channel of an established plaque. Once the wall ruptures, it starts to swell with blood. To form a plug over the top of this communication, the body mobilises the sticky cells, known as the platelets, and a series of proteins known as the clotting cascade is set in motion to form a protein mesh known as fibrin. The combination of fibrin and platelets is what forms the clot. The clot then plugs up the hole caused by the rupture, preventing any further blood from swelling the wall. If the clot is large enough (depending on the size of the rupture) it may completely block the artery, inducing a heart attack if the rupture occurs in the coronary arteries.

Certain individuals, however, through either genes or some environ-mental circumstances, have blood that is more prone to clotting. Many of these clotting disorders are not particularly rare and all it takes is the right sort of stimulus to set these clotting mechanisms into motion.

Case study: Joanne Walters—Joanne Walters is 62 years old. The day after she arrived in Sydney from Europe she noticed a swelling of her right leg. Her doctor examined the leg and felt, in view of the long plane trip, that Joanne was probably suffering a venous thrombosis (deep venous thrombosis or DVT). He started her on a course of warfarin (strong blood thinner). She remained on warfarin for three months and was then placed on Aspirin. The swelling and pain in her leg resolved and she returned to normal activities. Twelve months later she developed an acute episode of chest pain and was found to have had a moderate-sized heart attack involving the main artery in the front of the heart known as the left anterior descending. She recovered from the heart attack but was somewhat short of breath. She booked a CT scan of her coronary arteries, which showed a small speck of calcium in her left anterior descending, at the site of her prior heart attack. Her calcium score, however, was only 1, suggesting she had little in the way of atherosclerosis for a woman in her sixties.

On further assessment, Joanne had a normal cholesterol and normal blood pressure, had never smoked and had no family history of atherosclerotic disease. Her history was highly consistent with a pro-thrombotic state so I tested her blood and found that she had a relatively common condition known as antiphospholipid antibody syndrome. In many cases of anti-phospholipid antibody syndrome, the affected person should have lifelong warfarin therapy to prevent any further clotting episodes.

Even with minimal atherosclerosis, if you have a pro-thrombotic state, then your blood is thicker than the next guy's and rather than routine therapy with a drug like Aspirin, you may need more aggressive blood thinning with treatment such as warfarin.

There are numerous other causes of a pro-thrombotic state, which requires one blood test assessing for many different conditions. There are many genetic abnormalities that can thicken the blood. Suffice to say, I routinely screen for these blood disorders if I am given history of clots forming on either the arterial and/or the venous side of the circulation, or in someone that has little reason to have atherosclerotic disease but may have a personal or family history of thrombosis or emboli.

Cancer

Is this the most feared word on the planet? Despite the fact that many more women will die of some form of heart disease than breast cancer, if you polled a group of women in their forties, fifties or sixties, most of them would almost certainly say their greatest health fear is cancer, in particular, breast cancer. For most people, a diagnosis of cancer implies premature death preceded by either major surgery, radiotherapy or aggressive chemotherapy, or possibly a combination of two or three of the above. With early detection and better management of some cancers, orthodox medicine has reduced the death rates, but there does appear to be an increasing incidence of and still an ongoing carnage from this dreadful diagnosis.

In this modern era, when we can transmit information in the blink of an eye to any part of the globe, when we have designed computers with the power to store incredible amounts of information in such a small area, when we can bore tunnels through any piece of earth to redirect a major highway, we are still struggling to cure the common cold and have no definite explanation as to why people get cancer. There are numerous theories, from environmental poisons to genetic predisposition, and the rather novel and almost century-old argument of Dr John Beard that cancer is a deranged healing process in the body due to a lack of Vitamin B17, a deficiency of pancreatic enzymes and exposure to environmental toxins.

TYPES OF CANCER

What we do know for certain about cancer is that cancer cells are rapidly-growing cells with deranged metabolism that do not follow the normal rules of homeostasis and cell division. These cells have no respect for normal human tissue and hungrily steal nutrients from normal cells. There are numerous risk factors for cancer and it is worthwhile to consider some of the more common cancers and their associated risk factors.

Breast cancer

This very common cancer in women occurs for somewhere between one in five and one in 13 women during their lifetime, based on their own inherent risk factors. The strongest risk factor for breast cancer appears to be picking the wrong relatives. If your mother or sister had or has breast cancer, then your risk is probably around 20 per cent over your lifetime.

Although the evidence is not definitive, there appears to be a link between synthetic oestrogen and breast cancer. Unfortunately, many of the studies are conflicting and I believe the reason for this is that we are all different. Your oestrogen receptors respond differently to different types of oestrogen—one woman's oestrogen receptors are different to another's. In the case of hormone replacement therapy, I do not believe this causes breast cancer, but certainly if a woman has a predisposition to developing breast cancer, hormone replacement therapy may accelerate its growth.

There is no doubt that for women with severe peri-menopausal symptoms—such as flushing, fatigue, lack of libido, mood swings and irritability—hormone replacement has been a God-send. For other women, starting hormone replacement therapy signalled significant weight gain, nausea, headaches and a general downturn in quality of their life. The ability to induce or accelerate breast cancer, although only slight, has been shown in a number of studies and certainly hormone replacement therapy requires careful monitoring. There are very strong supporters of HRT and there are equally strong detractors. As with all aspects of prevention, I believe it is up to the individual to consider all of the evidence and their own personal risks before deciding on treatment.

Another theory of breast cancer causation is not using the body for what it was initially designed to do. Women usually undergo menarche (onset of periods) somewhere around the age of 11, up to the age of 14. The biological function of the female body is to procreate the species. In many traditional societies, women once became pregnant in their early teens and their mothers contributed significantly to the nurturing of the children. These days women are delaying having children until well into their thirties and sometimes early forties. Therefore, the uterus and the breasts are not being used for their intended function—growing an embryo and feeding the newborn baby.

If you do not use an organ as it was intended, it is believed this can cause all manner of bother. In the same way that we need to exercise our heart and muscles to achieve good health, women need to exercise their breasts and uterus in the way nature intended. There is, therefore, a relationship between the time from menarche to having your first child and your risk for breast cancer. Interestingly, there is a higher risk for uterine and breast cancer in nuns—probably for this very reason. There is also a higher risk for cervical cancer in prostitutes—probably for overuse of their cervix and vagina with multiple partners.

During the past many women felt that a blow to their breast could cause breast cancer. The only possible link here is that a blow to the breast can cause a haemorrhage in a tumour that is already present and therefore make the tumour easier to palpate. But a trauma cannot cause a tumour to appear. There is also no good relationship between the amount of children you have and your risk for breast cancer.

Lung cancer

It is stating the bleeding obvious to link cancer and cigarettes, but another interesting association is living in a city. If you smoke and are also exposed to excessive amounts of pollution, your risks for lung cancer are much higher than if you enjoy the tranquillity of a rural setting. I am not suggesting that smokers should pack up house and ship out to the country, but I strongly suggest that smokers make the decision to stop smoking . . . now! I often hear the argument from smokers about old granny who never smoked a cigarette in her life but developed lung cancer and died. Often when you press these people, old granny didn't smoke but old grandad was a heavy smoker and granny suffered the effects of side-stream or passive smoking.

There is also a much higher risk for lung cancer and other rarer cancers in workers in heavy industries, especially those exposed to asbestos.

Bowel cancer

Bowel cancer is an extremely common cancer and in almost all cases it affects the large bowel. With the advent of colonoscopy, many of these cancers are detected early. People who fear the diagnosis, however, sometimes foolishly avoid colonoscopies and other investigations, and wait until they present with symptoms. These symptoms can be anything from rectal bleeding to weight loss, fatigue and anaemia. A change in bowel habit or unexplained abdominal pain can also be a relatively common presentation.

The major risk factor for bowel cancer is having relatives with the same diagnosis. But genetics are quite difficult to assess. Often people born into the same family are brought up in the same environmental circumstances and continue with the habits of their parents as adults. It may be that the learned eating habits, which could certainly contribute to bowel cancer, are more cogent than a pure genetic predisposition.

There is some weak evidence linking lack of dietary fibre and increased risk for bowel cancer, but definite evidence exists linking a high intake of fruit and vegetables and a low risk for bowel cancer. There are two unusual, though not rare, conditions that markedly increase the risk for bowel cancer: ulcerative colitis and familial adeno-matous polyposis coli. If someone suffers ulcerative colitis they need regular colonoscopies as their risk for bowel cancer is around 17 times that of normal. Familial adenomatous polyposis coli has an almost 100 per cent risk for bowel cancer and needs very careful management and supervision by an expert gastroenterologist and colo-rectal surgeon.

Prostate cancer

This is a very common diagnosis, especially in older males. There are no major risk factors for prostate cancer, although some proposed mecha-nisms are a reduction in sexual function and, therefore, reduced use of the prostate gland. Chronic prostatic infections may also predispose to the eventual development of a prostate cancer. There is an inverse rela-tionship between the intake of lycopene through tomato-based foods. Cooked tomatoes, tomato paste and tomato sauce, especially, increase the lycopene content of the bloodstream, therefore decreasing the risk of prostate cancer.

Female genito-urinary cancers

The three common female genito-urinary cancers are cancer of the cervix, cancer of the uterus and cancer of the ovaries. Although cancer of the ovaries is not as common as the other two types of cancers, it is vital that females have regular monitoring to detect any signs of these cancers early on.

CONTROVERSIES IN TREATMENT

Over the past 30 years we have seen a vocal minority claim they have been cured of this disease through non-traditional methods. These cures have been labelled as 'spontaneous remissions' by orthodox medicine. Traditional practitioners have stated that there is no explanation for them and they are completely unrelated to whatever techniques are being lauded by the so-called recipients of the cure. A number of these recipients have gone on to promote the cures, believing they have the answer to cancer or, possibly in some cases, to profit from their good fortune. Numerous people have often 'as a last resort' bundled themselves off to cancer clinics—the most famous being the Tijuana Clinics in Mexico—some benefiting, others meeting their demise.

In the 1950s, a biochemist by the name of Ernst Krebs discovered a substance he called Vitamin B17, otherwise known as Laetrile. Krebs and his followers (including Edward Griffin, a Californian journalist who wrote the book *World Without Cancer*) suggested that cancer was, in fact, a deficiency of Vitamin B17—a notion that is hotly disputed by the conservative medical world. Vitamin B17, or Laetrile, has been depleted from our highly refined Western diets. Krebs and his followers suggest that the so-called poisons said to precipitate cancer, such as cigarette smoke, pollution, excessive chemicals in our foods and environment, are purely triggers that expose the Vitamin B17 deficiency.

SOURCES OF VITAMIN B17

The seeds or kernels of apricots, apples, plums, cherries (and other members of the botanical family Rosaceae), along with millet, crushed linseed, cassava and bitter almonds.

Vitamin B17 contains large amounts of nitrilosides. The argument forwarded by Krebs and his followers is that the nitrilosides in these natural food sources are harmless to normal human cells. Each molecule of B17 contains one unit of cyanide and one unit of benzaldehyde and two glucose molecules combined in a stable structure. An enzyme in cancer cells, known as beta-glucosidase, breaks the Vitamin B17 into cyanide and benzaldehyde within the malignant cell, causing rapid malignant cell death. The body contains another enzyme known as rhodanase, which overrides the enzyme beta-glucosidase in healthy tissues, thus preventing the breakdown of cyanide and benzaldehyde into a form that can damage the body.

Many years ago, millet and linseed bread was our major staple. These are rich sources of Vitamin B17. When we switched to wheat, a much cheaper alternative, we lost this rich source of Vitamin B17 and cancer presented itself as a problem in our community. The problem has sky-rocketed over the past 20 to 30 years because of our increasing dependency on technology and the toxic by-products of this dependency. Edwin Griffin argues in his book that some communities, such as the Hunzas in Pakistan, allegedly never developed cancer. Their diet is very high in apricot kernels and millet. When the Hunzas became more exposed to Western society and started to adopt more of a Western diet, their rates of cancer increased.

In December 2000, there was a report from London citing that mainstream researchers had used the cassava plant as a method for killing cancerous tumours in human beings. Basically, this is exactly the same product (i.e. Vitamin B17), that has been outlawed in many countries as a treatment for cancer. Mainstream medicine, however, states that Laetrile has been tested in at least 20 tumour models using isolated cancer cells or animals and has been found to have no benefit. Studies of case reports of humans have also been negative. Mainstream medicine states that Laetrile is not without side effects, and many cancer patients have reported nausea, vomiting, headache, cyanosis, fever, mental confusion, coma and dizziness—all symptoms of cyanide poisoning. (I must say, however, that some of these certainly sound like symptoms of chemotherapy as well.)

It is illegal to either import or sell the product in Australia, and the United States. I am neither deriding nor supporting this treatment, but I believe it is important for this information to be disseminated to the general public, to allow the intelligent consumer to decide. For those of you who are interested in exploring the subject, it is my advice that you look at both sides of the argument. The website against the use of Laetrile is <www.cancernet.nci.nih.gov/cam/laetrile.htm>. The website in support of the use of Laetrile is <http://geocities.com/vialls/index.html>.

Case study: Jason Winters—In 1977, at the age of 46, Sir Jason Winters developed an infiltrating squamous cell carcinoma affecting his carotid artery and jugular vein, manifesting initially as a swelling on the side of his neck. He underwent radiotherapy, which caused all sorts of side effects including loss of taste, inability to make saliva, and burning of the right side of his face. He then heard about the very controversial treatment known as Laetrile.

Supporters of Laetrile therapy believe it is important to take supplemental pancreatic enzymes as well as Vitamin B17. Jason Winters began the treatment with an initially superb response. Despite this, and despite taking 3000 mg of Laetrile every day as well as the pancreatic enzymes, his tumour returned. Not being someone to take things lying down, Jason travelled all around the world to find a cure for his cancer.

He tried a herb in Singapore known as herbalene, which had little effect. He kept the herb, and then travelled to Tucson, Arizona, where he drank a herbal tea known as Chaparral (from the creosote bush). Again, there was little effect from this preparation. When he returned to England he was told about red clover. This herb by itself had no real effect.

By this stage Jason had spent all of his money and was desperate, so he mixed the three herbs together. After doing this he started to feel better. Within a few days he was markedly improved and within a few weeks his tumour had shrunk. Sir Jason Winters has continued to use this herbal combination, along with some other interesting supplements and now, 25 years later, he travels the world telling his story and marketing his alleged cancer-curing preparations.

Mainstream medicine, however, has other explanations. Some quarters say that Winters never had cancer in the first place. Others say he did have cancer but that his cure was due to a spontaneous remission and the ingestion of useless herbs was pure coincidence. Another possible explanation is his extraordinary determination to fight the disease. Doctors love measurements and one of the things that we certainly cannot measure is attitude. Many people are on a self-destructive path and their cancer or heart disease is an inevitable consequence for the way they have lived. In this situation it makes it very difficult for them to muster any sort of willpower, fight, determination—call it what you will—to overcome such an incredible setback.

The medical paradigm for treating cancer is to cut out the tumour and radiate the offending area or poison the body with chemotherapy in the hope that the cancer cells will be killed and the body will recover. There is no doubt that many childhood leukaemias are cured by this approach, as are many lymphomas and some adult leukaemias. Testicular cancer, again, has a very good response to standard medical therapy.

Oncologists would agree, however, that once a solid tumour (such as a breast cancer, bowel cancer, lung cancer or prostate cancer) has spread away from the organ of its origin, then the survival rates on a long-term basis are rather dismal. This then brings up a very controversial question: are all the people across the world who are claiming cures with non-traditional medical approaches purely charlatans or do they have something to offer?

Medical science will claim they have researched these non-traditional treatments but in their studies have seen no real benefit from the treatments that the Laetrile proponents or the supporters of other non-traditional therapies have claimed to be miracle cures. The retort from the supporters of non-traditional cancer therapy is that the treatment was not used correctly by the researchers. For example, in the case of Laetrile, they did not combine Laetrile with pancreatic enzymes, nor did they use detoxification, which often involves the process of clearing out toxic substances—usually by using some form of enema.

The supporters of this type of detoxification use anything from oxygen to caffeine to clear the colon, ridding the body of the toxins spilling into our circulation, causing all manner of ills. This concept is totally rejected by orthodox medicine, but in many quarters of complementary medicine, it is very much embraced. Do these people have some form of magical purification process or are they just a bunch of anally retentive individuals who are obsessed with their colons? My answer to this is very frank and honest: I don't know! Between you and me, I prefer my coffee by the normal route, and with my rather vigorous consumption of fruit and vegetables and unprocessed bran, I suspect I'm doing a perfectly good job of detoxifying my colon by these methods.

In defence of science, most people working in the field are trying their best to be objective and use the scientific methods. Many of the methods used by alternative practitioners do lack the scientific control demanded by the rigorous conservative scientific bodies, but I can still appreciate and, in many ways, sympathise with the cynicism increasing among the general public regarding the authorities either in science, medicine or the general administration of our society.

Many people will go to great lengths to hold on to power and there is no doubt that industries such as the cancer industry or what I loosely call 'the chest pain industry' are in a very strong position of not only emotional power, but also financial power in our community. Many multinational groups, institutions and organisations are making billions of dollars out of sick people. It is also important, however, to realise that the pharmaceutical industry has developed thousands of very sophisticated medications that have, in many cases, prolonged people's lives. I must state as well that, having been through the training, most of the people I have worked with and trained with over the years have been extremely dedicated, caring people. I am the first to admit that many lack bedside manner, but it is a small minority that lack compassion and only view the practice as purely a money-making exercise.

I don't have an answer to these conflicting claims, but I can certainly give you some guidelines as to what I would do if I was ever diagnosed with a cancer. If it was a hematologic cancer, such as leukaemia, lymphoma or a testicular cancer, I would not hesitate to undergo conventional therapy for this condition. At the same time, however, I would be obtaining as many natural sources of Vitamin B17 as possible, along with the use of pancreatic enzymes, and drinking Sir Jason's herbal tea preparation. If I had a localised bowel cancer, again, I would not hesitate to have this surgically removed as the cure rates for early colon cancer with limited or no spread are close to 100 per cent. If, however, I developed any solid tumours (such as all the common cancers) that had spread beyond their initial site, I would plunge myself into nutritional therapy and certainly not bother with any form of chemotherapy, radiotherapy or surgery. This would be my personal decision and it is certainly not a medical recommendation; but I'm not entirely sure that most members of the profession would disagree.

One thing we haven't discussed, which is again certainly controversial, is the psychological aspects of cancer. Is cancer purely bad luck due to a mixture of environmental toxins and poor genetics? Is it, as many people in the alternative world believe, a nutritional deficiency due to varying low levels of different types of natural chemicals (such as Vitamin B17)? Or is cancer possibly due to a more profound but little discussed issue?

A woman called Caroline Myss has written some excellent books, including *Anatomy of the Spirit* and *Sacred Contracts*. She firmly believes (and I must say that I don't totally disagree) that all illnesses have a psycho–spiritual basis. In her books, she discusses the seven Hindu chakras, the seven Christian sacraments and the 10 Jewish sefirots. She says these represent energy areas or centres within the body and, depending on your progression through life's journey, will determine where your illnesses occur. The seven energy areas are:

1. Relationship to the tribe: The first centre concerns how we interact in our immediate and global community, our connection to our family and our friends, and generally how we are perceived. If you have a problem in any of these areas, this can often manifest as problems with your immunity or problems with your lower back and musculo–skeletal system. This energy centre is located at the bottom of your spine. Basically, you're sitting on it.

2. Our relationship with others: This centre basically reflects on your ability to have sound interpersonal elationships. If you have problems with, or are struggling with power over other people, this can manifest as diseases in your sexual organs, or problems with sexual function. It can also represent lower colonic problems. This energy centre is located around and just below the belly button.

3. Intra-personal problems: Your ability to understand yourself and to achieve some degree of self-awareness and knowledge is covered here. Problems in this area manifest as upper-gastrointestinal problems, such as problems with ulcers, reflux and gall bladder disease. This is located in the centre of the solar plexus.
4. Our emotional centre: This is the centre of unconditional love and concerns problems in the central chest area. It reflects our ability to give or receive unconditional love and manifests as heart problems, blood pressure or breast cancer.
5. Our decision or choice centre: This is located around the throat. Conditions in this area include thyroid abnormality, recurrent sore throats and cancers of the head and neck.
6. 'The third eye': Located in the centre of the forehead just above the level of the eyes, this is the centre of intuition and knowledge. Problems in this area can be manifested as headaches, stroke or, more concerning, brain tumours.
7. The crown: Located on the top of the head, this is our direct connection to God.

Many conservative people reading this will think this is completely 'whacko'. Those with a more open mind will find it very interesting, but I still believe it is important to be sceptical and ask questions. From a medical viewpoint, I often find people who I would consider to be stuck in one of these areas and they *do* tend to have conditions related to this particular energy centre. Is there any real value to this? Possibly.

Caroline Myss argues very strongly that women who develop breast cancer have one of two problems. The first is that they are either excessive nurturers in that they give all of their self to their families or to their husbands and they don't particularly spend much time on themselves. I believe it is important that people put effort into their own health and into their own life. Having time for your own interests and for self-nurturing allows you to be a more rounded person. I certainly don't mean to suggest that anyone who is a wonderful nurturer of children or is a very devoted wife will end up with breast cancer. But in my experience most women (certainly not *all*) who develop breast cancer do so at a stressful time in their life. Often, breast cancer arises around the time of a marriage break-up, the death of a parent, or some significant life change. A more objective person may argue, however, that the occurrence of the cancer altered the person's perception of their life and made them believe that their marriage was going badly, they were very unhappy, or whatever situation they are alluding to.

The other interesting suggestion Myss argues regarding breast cancer is the other extreme—the non-nurturing types. These are women who do not want to have children and are so obsessed with themselves that they are, in many ways, selfish. It is the person who may not be using their breasts for what they were intended—feeding someone else.

These theories are very interesting and may have some credence, but also, many people reading this book might find them utterly offensive. Let me state right now that none of these are my ideas—I am just presenting the different controversies and allowing you to make up your own mind.

With prostate cancer, Caroline Myss believes that men who develop this have lost their power. It often occurs in older men who have retired, but also in men who once were prominent but now perceive themselves to be less important.

Case study: Adam Peale—Adam Peale is a 49-year-old vice-president of a software company. He was always a very ambitious man who rose to his position in the company very rapidly and was soon to take over as president. He had been married for 22 years and had three children, the oldest being 16. He was never what one would call a dedicated father and left most of the parenting to his wife. He certainly spent more time concerning himself with matters related to the company than he did with family issues.

When Adam was 44 he started having an affair with a 32-year-old marketing executive in the company. Although this was common knowledge throughout the office, he kept his secret carefully guarded from his family. As he was travelling on a regular basis, he could easily manage his secret liaisons without arousing his wife's suspicions. As with all these situations, however, Adam's misdemeanours were eventually discovered by his family. One of his wife's friends saw him dining with his girlfriend and felt it her duty to tell his wife. The affair had been in progress for over two years and Adam felt he was in love with his co-worker. He confessed all to his wife and decided to leave home.

When the relationship became common knowledge in the company, the board of directors frowned on Adam's behaviour and he was demoted. He married his girlfriend but she was an extremely ambitious and controlling person and not particularly happy with Adam's demotion. She let him know in no uncertain terms.

Adam was feeling rather tired with some aches in his lower back and made an appointment with his doctor for a check-up. The doctor ran some tests, including a PSA (prostate specific antigen), which showed a very high level. Adam was referred to a urologist and a diagnosis of prostate cancer was made.

Was this a coincidence or was it due to Adam's loss of power over his life?

There are many theories also regarding the true cause of heart disease. Is heart disease purely a compilation of many risk factors or is there a strong psycho–spiritual component? Certainly people like Caroline Myss believe so, and there has been much work done regarding different personality characteristics, such as the type-A and type-B people. There is no doubt from the literature that there is a strong association between the hostile, time-urgent, angry person and heart disease. It is this person that Myss would say has problems at their fourth energy level. Who knows, all of our illnesses may be just pure bad luck, but I suspect this is not the case.

One of the areas that really does need to be explored in terms of not just recognition of a problem, but also treatment, is that of the use of meditation and visualisation in people with serious disease. There have been quite a number of case reports of people with cancer who have spent up to one hour a day developing a meditative state to visualise situations that will change the orientation of their cancer.

For example, I had one patient who had a diagnosis of secondary prostate cancer. Every day for one hour he would lie in a comfortable position on the floor and imagine an army of ants were eating away at his cancer. After he had performed this unusual ritual for around two or three months, he was shown to be free of cancer by his doctors. Another young boy with a brain tumour visualised that he was Luke Skywalker in his spacecraft firing at the tumour and pulverising it out of existence. Again, this young boy was declared cured of cancer. Are these purely 'spontaneous remissions' or does the visualisation have something to do with the cure?

Case study: Ian Gawler—In the 1970s, a psychiatrist in Melbourne known as Ainslie Meares reported a type of meditation known as atavistic regression. This involved taking your psyche back to a time long before you had developed cancer. One of his devoted students was a man by the name of Ian Gawler. Ian had a condition known as osteogenic sarcoma. (Movie buffs will remember the movie *Sunshine*—the theme song was sung by John Denver—where the leading lady had the same condition.) Ian Gawler lost his leg and the cancer spread throughout his lungs. He was told he only had a few weeks to live. Using the techniques taught to him by Professor Meares, within a few weeks he had improved and is still alive today, running clinics in Victoria where he teaches people the importance of meditation, a positive mental attitude and nutrition.

A friend and colleague of mine, Petrea King, had a diagnosis of terminal cancer made 20 years ago during a very traumatic period in her life. Petrea travelled to Italy and meditated for hours on end in the cave said to have been visited frequently by St Francis of Assisi. Petrea was later cleared of any traces of cancer. Maybe visualisation and meditation work. Maybe they don't. I personally have been meditating for over eight years and can attest to the power of meditation as a technique to induce wonderful peace and calm. Does it cure cancer? Again, I don't know. Do I suggest you meditate? Absolutely!

Another large area of treatment controversy is that of chelation therapy, a treatment of poisoning by lead or other heavy metals with chelating agents. There are intravenous chelation services and some drugs that are said to act as oral chelation agents. One of the interesting aspects of chelation therapy is that it involves a strong nutritional program that encompasses antioxidant therapy and good nutrition. This begs the question: is it just this component of the total package that works or is there some benefit from chelation? If you believe the most recent trial, which appeared to be quite well conducted, there is no benefit. A recent large study from Canada, which was a randomised, controlled, blinded study of chelation in coronary artery disease, showed absolutely no benefit from chelation therapy. Intravenous chelation is very expensive, whereas oral chelation requires long-term ingestion of the medications.

Personally, with CT scanning of the coronary arteries, I have seen some people who appear to have benefited significantly from chelation and other people who have had no response whatsoever. Again, having contact with quite a number of doctors who work in the field of chelation, I know them to be dedicated professional people who are not charlatans or snake-oil salesmen. I also know that many of their patients appear to have benefited from their therapy. Can I write that I agree or disagree with chelation therapy? It is a controversial area and it is my suspicion that some people do respond well but many don't.

It is exactly the same principle as used for Laetrile, the difference being that the scientists involved can't patent this treatment and make a lot of money. Although people like to complain about these dreadful multi-nationals, they are also very happy to embrace all of their products, created for our convenience, comfort and entertainment. It is a modern-day dilemma. No longer should you accept everything that you are told by authorities. By all means, listen to experts but research the topic for yourself. The information is all there, it is no longer kept within the sanctity of some medical institution or government office. The only strong piece of advice I can give you is this: whenever you are faced with a particular dilemma or question, look at both sides of the argument, because the answer is probably somewhere in the middle.

Insulin resistance

When humans first crawled out of the primeval slime in an attempt to gain a bit of sophistication, we initially consumed a high-carbohydrate diet to feed two very strong, evolutionary organs—the brain and the reproductive tissues. We required glucose as our major fuel. We eventually evolved to be more suited to a high-protein, low-carbohydrate diet. Despite the low-carbohydrate intake, it was still important for the brain and the reproductive organs to have a steady supply of glucose. One of the mechanisms the body developed to cope with this was to become insulin-resistant. Being insulin-resistant stops the sugar from getting into the cell and runs the blood sugar level slightly higher. This is, therefore, an evolutionary advantage if you are a hunter–gatherer, living a life that is pretty much feast-and-famine, as you could consume plenty of glucose when it was available.

These days, however, the only hunter–gathering we do is hop into our cars and drive down to the local supermarket, pick up our supplies and drive back home. By and large, our life is an ongoing feast. Natural selection would therefore result in a high proportion of people who were insulin-resistant—those who were more insulin-sensitive would not have responded well to the high-protein, low-carbohydrate diet of today. Inhabitants of areas that were geographically isolated for thousands of years, such as the Pima Indians in Arizona, could therefore have possibly evolved quite significant resistance to the effects of insulin, which would have held them in good stead for their typical native diet. Unfortunately, when this group of people were exposed to Western diets, their bodies could not cope and the consequences have been disastrous.

Interestingly, the Europeans have the lowest rates of insulin resistance and it is felt that this is because they were the first to be exposed (at least 10 000 years ago) to agriculture with a diet relatively high in carbohydrates. In fact, the rates of insulin resistance among Caucasians are around 30 per cent, among Asians probably in the 50–60 per cent range, with varying degrees of insulin resistance present in almost all people of black extraction. This is why many Maoris, Aboriginals and South Pacific Islanders appear heavier than their Caucasian counterparts.

In 1988, Professor Gerald Reaven first introduced the term 'Syndrome-X'. It is probably better described as insulin resistance. Insulin resistance may be purely genetic or there could be an environmental component. For example, obese people appear to be quite insulin resistant. Is it the obesity that causes the insulin resistance, or the insulin resistance that causes obesity? At this stage, no-one is really sure whether it is the chicken or the egg. Suffice to say, it is an increasing problem, so much so that it's becoming the Western epidemic of the new millennium.

The big question is what causes it in the first place. I have no doubt there is a genetic component, but until we have gene therapy and better genetic testing, whether it is genetic or environmental is rather irrelevant. The only means we have of dealing with this condition at present are environmental.

I believe insulin resistance occurs in the following sequence. Exposure to synthetic, processed foods floods our bodies with trans fatty acids and processed carbohydrates. The trans fatty acids incorporate into the membrane or covering of the cells and the normal fluidity and permeability of these membranes is significantly affected. The cell wall thickens to make them more rigid and impermeable to substances. The protein receptors, which sit on the cell membrane, can no longer function normally. One of the major protein receptors is the glucose transporter. This glucose transporter requires insulin to allow glucose to be actively transported (using energy) into the cell where it is used as a nutrient. Because the receptor is not working normally, it becomes insensitive, or resistant, to the effects of insulin. Thus, the cell believes (correctly so) that it is being starved of one of its major energy supplies—glucose—therefore the body craves carbohydrates.

I don't know how often I hear people say, 'I get so hungry that I *must* have [a biscuit, a piece of cake, an ice cream, a piece of chocolate, a lolly]' or some other quick sugar fix, to restore their failing energy. I, therefore, feel one of the major ways to cope with insulin resistance is to reduce the intake of synthetic trans fatty acids and synthetic carbohydrates.

THE CONSEQUENCES OF INSULIN RESISTANCE

Diabetes

If you asked the man on the street, 'What is diabetes?', the most common answer would be: 'A lack of insulin from the pancreas.' In fact, less than 10 per cent of diabetics are what are known as 'insulin-dependent' diabetics. This is the usual diabetes of childhood. Without insulin, the blood sugar rapidly rises, the person commonly becomes extremely thirsty and they pass significant amounts of urine. Their fatigue levels increase and, if the diagnosis is not made quickly, the affected person will develop a condition known as diabetic ketoacidosis. Without urgent therapy, usually in a hospital, there is a chance of death. These people are insulin-dependent for the remainder of their lives and they often require up to four injections of insulin per day.

There has been some promising work with different types of pancreatic transplants. There is also significant work being done on inhaled forms of insulin. It is the hope of every insulin-dependent diabetic that at some stage in the near future, this form of diabetes will become a completely painless exercise—the blood sugar being monitored by a finger probe rather than recurrent finger-pricks, and the insulin being delivered via an inhalant rather than with an injection.

The most common form of diabetes, however, which is becoming the growing epidemic in our society, is non-insulin-dependent diabetes. Non-insulin-dependent diabetes is caused by an entirely different underlying pathology. It is felt that the most likely cause is insulin resistance. When a person is insulin-resistant, the constant bombardment of their cells with sugar requires more insulin to be released from the pancreas. After years of this cellular and pancreatic abuse, the pancreas starts to say, 'Forget it, fellas. I've had enough.' The pancreas, over-loaded with work after years of secreting more insulin than the body really can cope with, starts to fail and the blood sugar starts to rise.

Non-insulin-dependent diabetics also presents with marked thirst, the passing of significant amounts of urine, and fatigue, but they do not become ketoacidotic as they are still making adequate amounts of insulin to prevent this from occurring. In short, their blood sugar rises and they require treatment. Strangely enough, the best treatment for a non-insulin-dependent diabetic in the first instance is returning to a sensible diet and exercise program. Weight loss is vital.

The argument between different factions is whether this diet should be centred around an increase in complex carbohydrates and a reduction in saturated fat, or more a reduction in trans fatty acids, most forms of carbohydrate, with an increase in the good forms of fat and protein.

The standard treatment for non-insulin-dependent diabetes after diet and exercise is the use of drugs that improve insulin resistance, such as metformin. There is a new group of drugs known as the glitazones, which have a very specific and strong effect on improving insulin resistance. One of the mainstays of drug treatment are the sulphonyl ureas, but there is a problem with using these drugs in that they release more insulin from an already failing pancreas. This is almost like flogging an injured horse. But for most people, the choice is either using these drugs or proceeding straight to good old insulin via injections. Most, of course, prefer swallowing the pill rather than having to inject themselves a few times each day.

There is no argument in the medical world about the importance of glucose control. Persistent elevations of blood glucose cause all sorts of bother. One of the disastrous consequences of having too much of this sugar travelling around in your bloodstream is the formation of substances known as glycosylated end products (GEPs). What this basically means is the excess sugar gets stuck in the normal body proteins. For example, in our red cells there is a protein known as haemoglobin, which carries oxygen around the body within the red cells and deliver this oxygen to the tissues, where it is used in the mitochondria of our cells to create energy. A significant reduction in our haemoglobin concentration means there is not enough oxygen getting to the tissues.

As the red blood cells are accessible, we can use the glycosylation of haemoglobin as an indication of diabetic control. There is a test known as haemoglobin A1-C, which is an indication of how much glucose is flooding into the body. As the red cells survive in the body for around three months, a haemoglobin A1-C level is an excellent indication of three-month diabetic control because it gives a level of how much additional unwanted glucose is in the system.

The excessive glucose does not just affect the haemoglobin in red cells, it can also affect other vital body proteins such as LDL cholesterol and collagen. When the glucose floods these proteins it makes them more sticky and less able to perform their normal function.

Just because you may have a normal blood sugar level, it does not mean that the excessive sugar you may be taking in your diet is not causing issues within the body. It is felt that GEPs also occur in people with insulin resistance, even without diabetes being diagnosed. It certainly contributes to the numerous clinical syndromes occurring as a consequence of being insulin-resistant. Just imagine these GEPs as you would a lolly that has melted in your pocket. The next time you put your hand in your pocket you would feel the sticky, gluggy mess on your fingers and it would be very difficult to restore that pocket back to normal. This is quite analogous to the situation in your different body systems, and in particular, your blood vessels and other major tissues throughout the body.

Hypertension

Although I have stated that around 30 per cent of Caucasians are insulin-resistant, the figures for those suffering high blood pressure are probably more in the 60 to 70 per cent range. Insulin resistance is a major factor in the causation of high blood pressure and people who are diabetic require even lower blood pressures compared with the rest of the population. If your doctor finds your blood pressure is starting to rise, it is also very important to have tests for diabetes and cholesterol, and it is vital to keep your weight in the normal range.

Abnormal fat profile

When we talk of fat in our bloodstreams we usually think of high cholesterol. Unfortunately, as with most things in medicine, this is far too simplistic. It is my firm opinion—backed up by numerous scientific papers—that cholesterol, in many cases, is just an innocent bystander and more of a marker for other problems. This is especially so in the insulin resistance syndrome. People who are insulin resistant classically have a minor elevation in cholesterol, probably in the range of 5 to 6 millimoles per litre—although on some occasions even lower. More concerning, however, is a triglyceride level above 2 millimoles per litre and an HDL of 1 or less.

I was extremely disappointed the other day when I saw a patient who had been told by her diabetic specialist that her cholesterol levels were perfect. When I reviewed them her total cholesterol was 5, her triglycerides were 3 and her HDL was 0.9. These levels are far from perfect and, in fact, are very concerning. The combination of high triglycerides (anything above 1.5) and a low HDL (anything below 1.3) should immediately alert your doctor that you are at a higher risk for some sort of vascular event.

Obesity

There is no doubt that obesity is a growing problem in all developed countries. The easy access to foods, especially of the convenience variety, combined with reduced exercise, means that people are expanding at a great rate. Throw in the gene for insulin resistance with the associated higher insulin levels and these people are a walk-up start for obesity.

Insulin by itself prevents the breakdown of fat and very rapidly shifts glucose into triglyceride metabolism, which promotes the laying down of fat cells. Having the insulin-resistant gene does not give people an excuse to be overweight, but really means that they have to work much harder than the rest of the population to keep their weight controlled.

Glucose and free radicals

Excessive amounts of glucose very commonly auto-oxidise to become free radicals. Glucose is one of the most oxidisable chemicals and, when you add all the other synthetic garbage we are exposed to, it is not hard to understand why excessive levels of glucose in the body, and thus high levels of insulin with the insulin-resistant syndrome, can cause so many health problems.

All of the above problems combine to cause rampant vascular disease in people with the insulin resistance syndrome. The warning signs for insulin resistance are as follows:

1. Diabetes—this should be expanded to include even a person found to have a random elevation of blood sugar or a history of diabetes during pregnancy.
2. Elevated blood pressure.
3. An abnormal cholesterol profile—especially characterised by high triglycerides and low HDL (good cholesterol).
4. Obesity, especially abdominal obesity—what is described in males as a beer gut. Just think logically, if you have fat around your belly, it's probably clogging the arteries around your heart.

TREATMENTS FOR INSULIN RESISTANCE

If you are highly suspicious that you are an insulin-resistance sufferer, don't panic! There is so much that can be done for insulin resistance to ensure that instead of spending your life supporting cardiologists' and endocrinologist's income, you can actually negate this as a problem in your life.

First and foremost, become a disciple to Cell Factor principles. The principles and practices of Cell Factor nutrition are ideally geared to improve and, in many cases, negate the effects of insulin resistance. The principles and practices of Cell Factor nutrition, however, don't just involve the sensible eating program detailed in this book. They also involve a global lifestyle change. One of the major problems with diets, exercise programs or joining the gym is the finite nature of these programs. Many people see a diet as being for a few months or a gym program for a few weeks. If you want to be healthy lifelong, you must practice healthy lifestyle principles lifelong.

There are, however, many more 'tricks' to improve insulin resistance other than just lifestyle change. Let me state from the outset, however, these extra tricks are not to replace the practices of Cell Factor Therapy, which is the foundation of all preventative healthcare programs. This includes programs for the prevention of cardiovascular disease, cancer, osteoporosis, Alzheimer's disease as well as insulin resistance.

Supplements for insulin resistance
CHROMIUM

Chromium in a dose of somewhere between 200 and 1000 micrograms a day improves glucose delivery to cells and diminishes the effect of insulin resistance. In a study performed conjointly between the United States and China, glucose levels were stabilised after four months of therapy with chromium.

My suggested dose is to start at somewhere between 400 and 500 micrograms. If no improvement in glucose levels is found after three to four months, I would suggest pushing this to 1000 micrograms a day. This can be taken on a long-term basis with limited toxicity.

ALPHA LIPOIC ACID

A significant improvement in insulin resistance was found in 74 diabetic patients given 600 milligrams of alpha lipoic acid a day. Alpha lipoic acid is an important component of the mitochondria—the energy store of the cell.

VANADIUM
The mineral vanadium in the form of vanadyl sulphate is showing some promise, but certainly at this stage needs more study.

GINSENG
Ginseng in a dose of either 2 or 3 grams as a supplement or in the form of tea is also showing promise in the treatment of insulin resistance.

CINNAMON
A simple way to improve insulin resistance is to add one teaspoon of standard cinnamon powder to whatever you have for breakfast in the morning.

OMEGA-3 FATTY ACIDS
I will discuss the enormous benefits of the essential fatty acids, of which Omega-3 is a major component, in a later chapter; but suffice to say, this has also shown promise in the management of insulin resistance.

VITAMIN E
Vitamin E as an antioxidant can specifically work to reduce the free-radical attack and subsequent oxidation of glucose.

This is a comprehensive summary of the supplements available specifically for insulin resistance but I am in no way suggesting that you should be swallowing each and every one. As I believe Vitamin E should be used as a preventative in almost all people over the age of 35 in a dose of somewhere between 400 and 800 units taken each night, I would consider this a standard recommendation. Specifically then, an initial supplementation regimen for the insulin resistance syndrome would be to start with:

- Chromium: 400 to 500 micrograms daily
- ginseng: either in the form of supplementation as tea
- cinnamon powder.

Alpha lipoic acid will probably be an excellent adjunct but at this stage it is somewhat expensive and is not as well tested as chromium.

Little things called quality and quantity

This piece of equipment we call the human body really is a masterful bit of engineering. But the big question we often ask ourselves is: 'why does it seem to wear out well before the age of 100? In fact, as we age, quite a few unpleasant things happen. Our hair becomes thinner, our skin wrinkles, vision becomes impaired and our hearing deteriorates. Blood vessels either crumble or stiffen, popping holes or clogging with fat. We lose our intellectual sharpness and memory often fades. Our joints and bones wear away, our teeth fall out and our gums recede. Gee, that sounds like a lot to look forward to!

From a purely biological viewpoint the physical vessel within which we live is almost perfect. The aim for life is to have a system that can survive and reproduce itself at sexual maturity. For most of us, this is our late teens and early twenties, even though now, in our modern society, people are leaving it till much later to have children, which, in many ways, is fighting evolution. This was fine in the hunter–gatherer days when the average lifespan was in the 30- to 40-year range. Either some nasty bacteria, a dreadful accident or possibly attack from another predator would bring about their early demise. So the system needed to reach its sexual maturity early, rather than somewhere between the age of 50 and 70 when we had at least developed some wisdom and emotional maturity. By this stage, the chance of survival in the hunter–gatherer era would've been so minimal that the human race would have become extinct many thousands of years ago. Therefore, for great evolutionary sense, we have stuck with the biological system we have, and it is up to us to do the best we can with it.

The function of every human being is to survive and it is interesting how we do so much to ourselves in this modern era that goes against that survival. With the baby-boomers in the main positions of power in society, the major push is not just longevity, but also quality of life. With rapidly advancing technology, our creature comforts have reached an unparalleled high. These comforts are ensuring that our quality of life, in terms of convenience, is unparalleled in human history. But material comfort is not the only area we should be seeking quality. I believe there are five areas of life that need to be explored and balanced. These are:

1. health
2. relationships and emotions
3. leisure
4. financial situation
5. spiritual life.

Quality of health

I once performed a cardiac ultrasound on a 75-year-old man, one of the richest men in Australia. He had achieved wealth beyond most people's dreams but had also suffered a series of heart attacks. His heart disease was *so* bad that on the scanner his heart was almost not pumping. He was bed-bound and could not walk down to his letterbox to retrieve his daily mail or the newspaper. I know it is obvious, but where does all that wealth get you if you don't have health?

Just recently I saw a very successful lawyer in his late thirties. He has a young family and works 12- to 14-hour days, sometimes six days a week. He was already on blood pressure medications and his weight was increasing rapidly. He played tennis and football in his teens and twenties but was now so busy that he didn't have the time to exercise. When he arrived home at night he was so tired from his day's activities that he could only swallow down his evening meal, rest in front of the television, stumble off to bed and wake up in the morning and start again. No-one would question this man's ability to do his job, but one would strongly question his ability in the self-management department.

I must stress again that there is no magic pill, potion or surgical procedure that can rectify any of these problems. The quest for good health and for a quality in your health is a global-lifestyle approach—it basically covers everything I will be discussing in next chapters. The road to optimum health includes:

- a medical assessment to determine your risk for future health problems
- a nutritional plan, involving sensible eating, moderate alcohol consumption and a balanced nutritional supplement program
- a regular exercise and movement program
- quitting smoking
- an ongoing stress-management program.

Quality of relationships and emotions

The enormous pressure that teenagers are under these days to perform well in their final exams at high school, I believe, is ridiculous. Unfortunately, this exam result and the subsequent academic performance at university often determine who will be awarded the top jobs in society. Many of these high achievers, although reasonable in the IQ stakes, are sadly lacking in the EQ stakes. EQ, or emotional intelligence, is our ability to empathise, to understand, to basically get on with our friends, colleagues and loved ones.

Case study: Mary—I remember when a dear friend of mine, Mary, rang me to tell me she had become deaf in one ear. I advised her to have an MRI (magnetic resonance imaging) of her brain, which demonstrated a tumour known as an acoustic neuroma.

This is benign, though very serious. It can cause all sorts of problems with hearing and balance. I referred her to a brilliant colleague of mine, who removed the tumour. Although the operation was successful, Mary developed a complication: an infection travelled into her wound area and she developed a secondary meningitis.

When my wife and I visited her in hospital she was quite delirious. She needed a new intravenous line put in her arm for antibiotic therapy. The young resident came into the room and did not acknowledge my wife or myself. He hardly spoke a word to Mary while he put the tourniquet on her arm and tapped her hand to try and make one of the veins stand up for the intravenous line. Not once did he look at her face and not once did he see that where he was tapping was causing her enormous pain.

This young man had no idea I was a doctor, and I could not stand by and watch my friend suffer at this person's arrogant onslaught. I suggested to him that the particular vein he was trying to attack had already been used and was inflamed, causing Mary significant discomfort. I found a virginal vein on the other arm and suggested he try that one with some local anaesthetic. He was taken aback by my comments but proceeded to follow my instructions when he found out I was a senior cardiologist.

The point of this story is to lament the fact that medical schools are spitting out people who had been in the top 1 per cent in their final exams at high school but, although probably reasonably intelligent, many of them are sadly lacking in emotional intelligence. This is not something that is peculiar to medicine, but happens in many professions and jobs. We are very quick to teach children the basics of schooling but we are not teaching them to be effective human beings.

In his book *Emotional Intelligence*, Daniel Goldman reported on a study where they put a group of toddlers in a room. They said to each toddler, 'Here is a marshmallow and if you could wait till I come back, I'll give you another marshmallow. But if you want to have this marshmallow now, you will not get the second marshmallow when I come back.' Some toddlers could not wait and consumed the marshmallow immediately. Other toddlers, although very tempted, would close their eyes, look away and wait until the researcher returned.

The researchers then followed these toddlers for a further 15 years and found that those who could wait for the second marshmallow scored much higher in their school leaving exams and had fewer problems with crime, drug addition and integration into society. Simply put, the toddlers who could exhibit delayed gratification (and I must say, the researchers being able to wait 15 years to finish the study showed enormous delayed gratification) were much more successful people.

I believe one of the major problems in our society is that we want it all, and we want it now. We are not prepared to wait. We are not prepared to put in the bigger effort that will reap rewards later on. This is seen clearly with burgeoning credit card debts and the inability of the community to save money and make investments for the future.

We need to focus more on teaching young children and teenagers the importance of relationships and emotions, rather than on achieving in exams. Basically, most of our life is centred around relationships and emotions rather than these other artificial situations. Many of us are now lamenting the lack of manners, even at the simplest level of talking to someone on the telephone regarding a business matter. I even object when someone rings my house for one of my children and they don't introduce themselves. I believe this lacks courtesy. Simple things such as these should be taught by parents, and reinforced at schools.

These first impressions can make or break a business, or even make or break relationships.

One of the main reasons for our existence is, of course, to nurture and care for those who are special to us. It will not be the board of directors of your company who will be standing around your bed when you have the heart attack. They will not be the people crying at your funeral. Even at a medical level the effects of a strong nurturing relationship are very profound. Dr Dean Ornish, a Californian cardiologist working near San Francisco, performed a study that involved feeding rabbits a high-processed diet for three months to see if they developed heart disease. Dr Ornish was shocked to find that only half the rabbits developed disease. When he researched the situation further he found that his lab technician loved rabbits—at every opportunity, she would go to the cages she could reach and take out the rabbits, pat them and play with them. It became no surprise to Dr Ornish to learn it was the rabbits in the cages she could not reach that developed the severe heart disease. Unfortunately, in these days of child abuse and sexual harassment, we are losing the importance of non-sexual touching. Many old people in nursing homes crave some form of human physical contact.

It is interesting that people who are involved in a strong nurturing environment do show less disease. In one study, women suffering from breast cancer had double the survival rate if they were shown to have strong emotional support. The same is true for heart disease, where many trials have shown that situations such as depression or a sense of hopelessness are associated with high rates of heart disease and higher complication rates in those with existing heart disease.

We all know that when we are run-down or feel emotionally drained we are much more prone to developing simple illnesses such as viruses. It is vitally important to put the time and effort into the people around you. The most important people, of course, are your immediate family. I often say that if for some reason someone's life ends prematurely, at work they are replaced rather quickly. In the family, however, they can never be replaced—all the more reason to make sure you do everything you can to be around for as long as you can.

Quality of leisure

Although I have just stressed the importance of spending time with family, I also believe it is important to have your own time. So many people spend too long at work, and whatever time is left, they give to their family. At no time are they nurturing themselves. I believe it is important to have interests outside work and the family, whether those interests be sport, a regular massage, music or spending time enjoying the natural environment.

A good friend of mine, Jerry, who is a real character and an excellent general practitioner, usually would not miss a day without getting on his mountain bike and riding around the national parks in his area. I am sure this balanced approach to his life keeps him sane.

Quality of financial situation

In these days where we all demand the material creature comforts, there is one significant downside: it all costs money. Housing, food, transport, school fees (if you have children), clothing, insurance and just enjoying some of the simple pleasures of life, such as a cup of coffee or a movie, all costs money. It is so important not only to enjoy your work, but to ensure that you are making the money you earn work for you. I am in no way a financial expert, as my accountant and financial broker will tell you, but my advice is to take some control of your finances and to plan for the future. Don't do it all yourself, however, seek the advice of an expert.

One strong piece of advice I can give is that if you hate your job, I suspect the universe is trying to tell you something. Maybe you should be looking elsewhere for employment.

Quality of spiritual life

I am not talking here about religion, as it is certainly not my place to do so. However, you know what would happen if you took all the people who fell asleep in church and laid them end to end? They'd be a lot more comfortable!

On a serious note, I believe we all need a reason to get up in the morning. What are your deeper life goals? Have you ever *really* considered this question? We spend so much of our life being affected by what's happening in front of our eyes and not really going behind our eyes to examine our deepest inner thoughts and feelings.

One of the key spiritual concepts is service to others. Over the centuries the people who have made a real mark on society in a positive sense have been those people who have been servers: Mother Teresa, Mahatma Ghandi and many other unsung heroes who spend their time in community service and are often not recognised for their hard work. Spiritually, one of our major motivating forces is love. If we seek and display unconditional love we are truly achieving our highest goals.

Quantity of life

Through the ages, human beings have been obsessed with immortality. Back in the days of Plato, Socrates and Aristotle this was a major topic of discussion. The ancient alchemists were on a constant quest for the Philosopher's Stone, the quest for immortality.

The basic fear of every human being is the fear of death. But it fascinates me to see how much people do to themselves every day to contribute to a premature death. Conventional medical wisdom tells us that a lifespan beyond 120 years is close to impossible. There are small pockets of the world, such as the Hunza Valley in Pakistan and in areas of Georgia near Russia, whose people claim to live well up to the age of 130 or 140. In *The Guinness Book of Records* there is a man in China who claims to be 250 years old. The reality is, however, these people do not possess birth certificates.

The longest-living person ever who could produce a birth certificate was Jeanne-Louise Clament. She died at the age of 122 in Paris a few years back. At the age of 121, she recorded a rap song! At the age of 120—and I must state this fact is like putting a knife into a cardiologist's chest and twisting it—she gave up smoking because she said it was becoming too much of a habit!

The most recent estimates for average life span, however, in Western countries, is around 75 for men and 80 for women. There are obviously a few countries and areas where the life spans are higher such as Japan and Crete, and, certainly, in under-developed countries the lifespans are much lower. Before the turn of the last century, however, around 40 per cent of people living in Britain could not expect to live beyond their 35th birthday. In those days, accidents and infectious diseases were the big killers. In our modern world it is heart disease and cancer.

A frightening new statistic, however, is the third biggest killer in the United States and Australia: medical intervention. In America the average death rate is around 2 million people per year. Of this figure, just over 40 per cent are due to cardiovascular diseases and another 30 per cent to cancer. Somewhere between 80 000 and 100 000 deaths, however, are due to complications of surgical intervention, serious reactions to medical therapy and a much smaller percentage due to medical mistakes. The aim for the twenty-first century is, therefore, not only improved treatment for heart disease and cancer and to markedly reduce the problems associated with medical intervention but, more importantly, much earlier intervention to prevent all of these problems.

IS LONGEVITY ON ITS WAY?

There are scientists all over the world working on the problem of longevity. Already the life spans of worms and mice, through modifying single genes, have been extended by up to 70 or 80 per cent. The particular gene, which was changed by Professor Tom Johnson from Colorado University, blunted the damage caused by free radicals. It is fascinating that by altering a gene that improves the body's mechanisms to neutralise free radicals, Johnson was able to markedly extend the lifespan of rather simple worms. By way of comparison, the human being has around 1 trillion cells per body, whereas the worms used in this experiment have just under 1000 cells. And, despite the reduced number of cells, the worm still has 19 000 genes whereas we have somewhere from 30 000 to 100 000 genes.

Another approach is not gene therapy, but uses a group of drugs known as synthetic catalytic scavengers (SCS compounds). These molecules are very powerful antioxidants. One of the problems with simple antioxidants is that once they donate one of their electrons, they themselves become free radicals. In the case of SCSs, however, once one molecule reacts with a free radical, another SCS molecule is created and thus these chemicals are much more powerful. The use of SCS drugs in the worms increased their lifespan by close to 50 per cent.

The downside of preventing these diseases is that people will be living longer, but often without a greater quality of life. Not only should we be trying to solve the longevity mystery, but also what I could loosely call the 'wearing-out' mystery—or better still, the wearing-out *misery*. What is the point of living to the age of 120 if for 40 years you're battling things like arthritis, poor vision, immobility and possibly other more serious illnesses.

Two major concerns of ageing, especially for baby-boomers but for most other people as well, is that of declining sexual function and declining physical appearance. The use of sexual performance–enhancing drugs, such as Viagra and many of the spin-offs that are emerging from this research, and the explosion of cosmetic surgery procedures show clearly that we are demanding medical intervention to 'improve' our quality of life with our extended quantity of life.

A proven life-extension therapy is straightforward caloric restriction. Experiments have been performed demonstrating that calorie restriction in mice doubles their lifespan, but in reality, who wants to live like that? An engineer in the United States by the name of Michael Cooper has lived on a calorie-restricted diet for a number of years: he has almost no body fat and, although only in his early fifties, looks around 10 to 15 years older. He eats per day what most of us eat in one meal, feels constantly cold and lacks a significant amount of energy. Another great exponent of calorie restriction is Professor Roy Walford, who wrote the book *The 120-Year Diet*. Walford believes that with calorie restriction, people may live to the age of 140. Again, Professor Walford is extremely thin and probably looks at least 10 years older than his stated age of 76.

We may eat far too much food, but do we have to go to the other extreme of eating far too little food and supplementing with micronutrients? Eating is one of our pleasures and I believe we should continue to enjoy this pleasure, but of course, not to the point of digging our grave with our knife and fork.

Woody Allen once said, 'It's not that I'm afraid of death, it's just that I don't want to be there when it happens.' If you ask most people in their twenties or thirties, they would probably be happy to die somewhere in their sixties, seventies and maybe eighties. Most would not want to live beyond that time. In a recent poll of 79-year-olds, however, all of them stated that they were more than happy to have quite a few more years of life. Basically, when we hear the wings of the Angel of Death flapping around our ears, we're happy to avoid the call. So is longevity good luck or good management?

I have no doubt from my own practice of medicine, my extensive reading and my personal research that improved quality and quantity of life can be achieved in most cases by a combined approach of early detection of future risk and management of whatever risks manifest with the global-lifestyle program. Our modern-day existence does afford us many more years and improved quality of life; we are, however, subjecting ourselves to two major areas of concern. As we live in a more artificial, synthetic environment, we are being exposed to many more synthetic agents, which are gradually poisoning our body systems through the mechanisms I have described. And, with the increasing synthetic nature of our environment, we are becoming increasingly deficient in the natural chemicals that are vital for the normal function of our body. The longer we live, the more we are exposed to this combined poisoning–deficiency combination and, therefore, the greater the potential that our bodies will succumb to these insults by manifesting disease.

We must, therefore, develop strategies that will help fight this relentless progressing of ageing and predisposition to disease. This is the subject of the next part of the book, 'The Cell Factor's Optimum Health Lifestyle Program'.

PART II

The Cell Factor's
Optimum Health
Lifestyle Program

The five-point plan

I have a patient, Chris, who is one of the most intelligent people I have ever met. Chris is a big-wig in the finance world and has a fascination with all matters medical. One of his interests is in preventative medicine. I would be more than happy to admit that Chris' knowledge of preventative medicine is better than most doctors'. He often emails me the latest study on any particular subject that he thinks I might find interesting. Instead of a doctor–patient relationship, Chris and I have formed more of a partnership to keep him well.

It is my firm belief that doctors in this new millennium should be two things to their patients: we should be educators and servants. Too many people go to doctors and say: 'Please, Doctor, help me. Please give me the latest pill. Please do the latest surgical procedure. Please get me out of this mess that I have created for myself.' I believe your illness is your responsibility and the medical profession is just there to assist you. Once you start to see this fact and start to use it to your advantage, you are already on the way to achieving optimum health.

The standard, traditional medical model is the disease model. Basically, you feel lousy with some symptom or other. You go to the doctor complaining of that particular symptom. The doctor formulates an hypothesis and, depending on his or her opinion of the severity of the condition, runs a few tests to either confirm or deny the suspicions. If the tests are suggestive of a particular condition, you are administered a treatment, which may be (in most cases) drugs or surgery. Hopefully, within a reasonable specified time frame the condition will sort itself out. The more serious the disease, the more intensive the investigations and the stronger the therapy. For example, a sore throat for a few days may indicate a viral infection and a competent doctor would suggest paracetamol or Aspirin, rest and plenty of fluids. Those health professionals with a more complementary bent will suggest, possibly, some Vitamin C, echinacea or zinc supplement. Severe central chest pain, however, may indicate coronary artery disease and, in particular, either unstable angina or a pending heart attack. Thus, more aggressive therapy, possibly even culminating in bypass surgery, is recommended.

Regardless of the diagnosis, that is what is known as 'the disease model'. This is a sound and effective way of treating a broad spectrum of diseases. Most diseases, however, are preventable—especially if the factors that caused them in the first place can be detected early and managed. This 'prevention model' is obviously a far more effective way of approaching health problems and saves the community enormous amounts of money. The prevention approach really is the way of the future and should be the major focus of health professionals—unless of course, you generate most of your income from people being sick! Many people give lip service to prevention but not many are pushing its barrow.

In this day and age, prevention is something that is very hard to sell. People are so used to instant answers and instant gratification that strategies requiring personal responsibility and a lot more effort on the part of the individual really do not fit into the modern notion of living. I have pointed the finger at the authorities, now I am pointing the finger at you.

One of the problems with prevention is that its results are hidden or not seen. If you line up a whole lot of people at high risk for a disease process, those at high risk will probably have a greater than 20 per cent chance over 10 years of developing that disease. From an optimist's viewpoint, this is less than an 80 per cent chance of *not* developing the disease. So if they all maintain the high-risk factors that promote the disease, after 10 years around one in five will have the problem. If you had brought in preventative strategies and nothing happens, it may not have happened regardless of the preventative strategies. Mind you, the longer you continue the preventative strategies, the closer the figure of nothing happening comes to 100 per cent.

The prevention model improves the safety rails at the top of the cliff rather than having the ambulance parked at the bottom to pick up the people who have slipped over the side. Unfortunately, our medical system treats most people only in the last five to 10 years of their life. Eighty per cent of the health dollar is spent on this group, obviously because they are the sickest and require the most intensive treatment.

Cost is a major issue for preventative medicine. Does the cost of preventative screening programs justify those detected of being at high risk? Who should pay for these preventative screening programs? Should it be the government, should it be health insurers? My opinion is that it should be paid for by the individual and probably by health insurance companies. I do not believe it should be a government responsibility. I do not believe people should be forced or coerced into having preventative health screens. If people are prepared to pay for something, they attach value to the service. If you are given something for free, it usually does not have the same impact. It is also my experience that people who are quite happy to pay for a high-quality preventative health service are the ones most likely to make the necessary changes to reduce their risk for any particular disease and, therefore, improve their health and longevity.

This part of the book will explain to you how to rectify the wrongs and prevent disease. It is never too late to repair any of the damage that has been done to your body. So, my very strong advice to you is to reclaim yourself, reclaim your body . . . because if you don't, no-one else will.

And the solution is not all that difficult. I have devised a five-point plan to help you achieve your optimum celluar health. It includes:

1. a baseline medical assessment
2. follow basic nutrional steps
3. regular, moderate exercise
4. quitting smoking (if applicable)
5. a daily program to manage stress.

Each person is different and you will need to adjust your lifestyle accordingly to fit the plan. For example, if you are already a non-smoker but do not exercise, then you will need to concentrate on the exercise component of the plan more than the smoking one. However, you will still need to understand the smoking component because 'passive' smoking has been proven to be harmful to cellular health.

The first step is a full base line medical assessment.

Have a baseline medical assessment

With all this talk about prevention and with preventative health assessments popping up all over the place, it is important to ask yourself who should be screened, when they should be screened and what level of screening should take place? An obvious answer to all of these questions is that screening should be performed on a need-to basis, based on a perceived or real notion of risk.

As a general rule of thumb, adults below the age of 35 with parents and first-degree relatives still alive and beyond the age of 65 do not require intensive screening programs. A relatively regular check of blood pressure, weight, simple urine testing and very occasional assessments of cholesterol and blood sugar are probably all that is necessary. For males above 40 and females above 50, however, I believe it is a different matter, and at this age I would suggest more intensive screening.

A preventative screen for all of the common diseases that may afflict us should follow these five basic strategies:

1. a careful history
2. physical examination

3 comprehensive blood testing
4. appropriate medical imaging
5. other tests when deemed necessary.

History
Your doctor should ask you about the following:

- Any current symptoms, such as chest pain, shortness of breath, dizziness, palpitations (sensation of the heart beating), cough (productive or non-productive), change in bowel habit, bleeding from any area, urinary symptoms, vaginal bleeding, breast lumps, etc.
- Risk-factor profile, involving such items as a history of cholesterol problems, high blood pressure, cigarette smoking, diabetes, alcohol consumption and other physical and behavioural factors.
- Past medical history, such as any prior history of all forms of heart disease, cancer, tendency to fractures and a full operation history.
- A full, comprehensive family medical history, including questions about diseases in parents, grandparents, siblings and other relatives. The age your family member was when they suffered a disease is very important. An older brother having bypass surgery in his forties is more relevant than a maternal uncle having a bowel cancer operation at the age of 75.
- A medication and supplement history, including social history and history of allergies.

Physical examination
A physical exam should include a general inspection of the skin assessing for any evidence of skin cancers or other skin diseases. It should also involve a thorough assessment of all pulses and a close examination of the heart and lungs with a stethoscope. The abdomen should be felt for lumps and enlargement of the liver or spleen, along with checks for hernia and abdominal aneurysm. A rectal examination should be performed for males, and for females an assessment for breast lumps and a pap smear should be done. A routine urinalysis

looking for sugar and protein should also be considered as part of every physical examination.

A blood test

I would advise these baseline blood tests: cholesterol, triglycerides, HDL, blood sugar level, uric acid, lipoprotein(a), homocysteine, highly sensitive C-reactive protein and apolipoproteins B and A1. I would suggest a haemoglobin A1-C level test, and some people may even want to go as far as having their fasting insulin levels measured. Ideal levels are as follows:

- If you have no evidence of significant vascular disease, total cholesterol should be less than 5 with LDL being less than 3. With evidence of vascular disease you should be aiming for a total cholesterol of less than 4 and an LDL level less than 2.
- Triglycerides should be less than 1.5.
- HDL should be greater than 1.3.
- Cholesterol–HDL ratio should be less than 3.5.
- Fasting insulin levels should be less than 10 millimoles per litre (any figures greater than 15 millimoles per litre indicates excessive amounts of serum insulin).
- Haemoglobin A1-C should ideally be less than 5 per cent (a figure of between 8 and 11 per cent is an indication of excessive amounts of glucose in the body).
- A good surrogate marker for serum insulin is the triglyceride–HDL ratio. Ideally this should be less than 1; 2 to 4 is concerning; greater than 4 is very high.

Some labs also perform assessments of electrolytes, and kidney and liver function, along with the blood count. Many doctors also believe that the performance of a PSA (prostate specific antigen) is an excellent screening test for cancer of the prostate. Other doctors argue that it is too sensitive and causes undue concern in the people with modest elevations. A normal result, however, suggests that the likelihood of a prostate cancer being present is extremely low.

Medical imaging

As a diagnostic procedure for disease, no-one would argue that CT (computerised tomography) scanning and MRI (magnetic resonance imaging) haven't revolutionised diagnostic radiology. There is, however, enormous controversy regarding the place of these, especially CT scanning, as a diagnostic screen for early disease. In the United States it is now common to have whole-body imaging as a screening test for disease. There are many supporters, but equally many detractors of these techniques.

The detractors suggest that there have not been enough long-term studies to support their general use. They argue that having your heart screened creates concern if the level is abnormal, and they also suggests that no-one really knows what to do with a high score. The supporters of this technique (and it is obvious that I am certainly one of these) are more than happy to refute these statements.

CT scanning of the coronary arteries detects calcium deposits within the arterial wall. The coronary arteries supply blood to the heart muscle and any sudden blockages within these arteries leads to heart attack and sudden cardiac death. Around one in four people in Western society will die this way, therefore it is very valuable to detect the process in its early stages. There are now well over 300 studies in the peer-reviewed medical literature supporting the use of coronary calcium scanning as a valuable technique for the detection of atherosclerotic coronary disease.

Coronary calcium scoring does not detect blockages in the arteries, it detects the process, sometimes decades before a blockage will occur. The newer machines, such as the multi-slice helical CT scanner—which rotates around the person at very high speeds, taking pictures of the heart in between heartbeats—can also detect fatty plaques without calcium. At this stage, however, a score of the non-calcium plaques cannot be given. Coronary calcium scoring itself is closely related to the amount of atheroscleroses (fatty build-up) present within the coronary arteries. There are numerous studies showing a direct correlation with the amount of coronary calcium, especially when matched to people of the same age, and your degree of risk for a heart attack or sudden cardiac death.

A recent study (see the *Journal of the American College of Cardiology*, 16 January 2002) showed that people with a score above 1000 had a 25 per cent yearly event rate. This is much higher than the event rate predicted from having high cholesterol, high blood pressure, or being a cigarette smoker, which has above a 20 per cent 10-year event rate. We consider, in general, scores above 400 for people over the age of 50 as being quite serious. A score of 100 to 400 is in the moderate range and 1 to 100 is considered mild. Any score in the 35–45 age range, however, should be considered as significant and the person should be followed carefully. Interestingly, in many cases we have been able to stabilise, and in quite a few, reverse the disease process with aggressive medical therapy. As a competition soccer player in my mid-forties, who still plays squash against his 23-year-old son, I was delighted to know I had a zero score, suggesting my risk over the next five years is extremely low.

It is my strong belief that males over 40 and females over 50 should have CT scanning of the coronaries as a matter of course, at least once. The only justification I can see for performing CT scanning below this age is if the person has a very obvious risk factor for premature heart disease, such as a first-degree relative with a history of vascular disease below the age of 55 or extremes of cholesterol abnormalities. Of course, long-standing diabetes also places a person at enormous risk for early vascular disease. Therefore, a special case would be a 35-year-old, insulin-dependent diabetic since the age of around 10.

Case study: Brian—Brian is a 55-year-old man who visited his general practitioner complaining of left elbow pain. His doctor reassured him that it was muscular and nothing to be concerned about. Brian wasn't very happy with this explanation as he had not been feeling particularly well. He attended my clinic for a CT scan.

Brian's score was 3000. Because of this I performed an urgent stress echocardiogram. After five minutes of gentle exercise on a treadmill Brian's left elbow pain occurred, his electrocardiogram changed dramatically and the whole front wall of his heart was moving the wrong way at the end of exercise. I have performed over 15 000 stress echocardiograms and this was the worst I had ever seen. I told Brian he was going straight to the hospital.

We admitted Brian and an angiogram was performed. This showed a 90 per cent block in his left main coronary artery, a 100 per cent block in the left anterior, descending 1 centimetre down the artery, and severe disease in the remaining two blood vessels—the circumflex and the right coronary arteries. Brian was a walking time bomb and needed urgent coronary artery bypass surgery.

After his bypass, Brian recovered very well. On further testing it was clear that he had high levels of lipoprotein(a). With his excellent bypass procedure and aggressive management of his underlying atherosclerotic process, including specific treatment directed towards lipoprotein(a), Brian is now doing extremely well.

Many critics of CT scanning say, 'The radiation dose of CT isn't worth the risk.' Well, what is the radiation dose from CT scanning? The average background radiation in our environment is around 300 milli-rems per year. One chest X-ray is around 50 millirems. A mammogram is around 500 millirems per breast (depending on the size of the breasts). A coronary angiogram can be anything from 30 to 100 times that of a standard chest X-ray. A CT scan of the coronaries is somewhere around 200 millirems and a full CT of the chest is 500 millirems. There-fore, the radiation dose from CT scanning is relatively low, and there has never been a reported case of cancer from diagnostic or screening radiation—*ever*. In fact, the degree of radiation from one CT of the coronaries would be equivalent to sitting in the window seat of an aero-plane for a few hours.

Many people ask, 'What about MRI?' Although MRI gives superb image quality, it is much more expensive than CT scanning and, certainly for the detection of coronary artery disease, still has some way to go. One of the other problems with MRI is the older scanners: they enclose the patient and many people are quite claustrophobic. This problem has been largely overcome by the open MRIs.

THE VALUE OF CT SCANNING

Screening for coronary artery disease is not the only value of CT scanning. A few years ago I was lecturing in Las Vagas to a large insurance group. A 48-year-old lady came up after my lecture wanting to talk privately to me about her medical problems. At first glance I saw a young-looking woman in her late forties, who appeared perfectly fit.

She told me that she had stopped smoking 15 months previously, concerned by the fact that both of her parents had died of lung cancer. Her astute physician suggested she undergo a CT scan of her lungs. This was despite a completely normal chest X-ray. The CT revealed two small, malignant tumours that had not, as yet, spread. The woman had part of her lung removed and the surgeon has given her the 'all clear'.

If her doctors had waited until a mass appeared on her chest X-ray, it probably would have been far too late. Now this lady is cured of lung cancer because of an excellent screening test. While CT scanning as a screen for lung cancer is in its early phases, you can adopt a conservative view of waiting until all of the scientific papers have been published. In the meantime, how many people will die from lung cancer until the science satisfies the medical profession?

Screening for gastrointestinal cancers is also a potential use with CT. Another exciting prospect is that of virtual colonoscopy. Although the best way to assess for bowel cancer is still colonoscopy, virtual colonoscopy is improving by the year, and I believe that in the next few years it will be a standard clinical screening assessment.

Other tests

The fifth area of preventative screening is more specialised tests. Tests in this category include **bone densitometry**. Osteoporosis is a significant and increasing problem in our community. The earlier this is detected and managed, the fewer problems will occur in later life. A hip or wrist facture can be a devastating problem, turning someone from an independent, mobile individual to a dependent, disabled person.

Carotid ultrasound is an excellent way of assessing the degree of carotid atherosclerosis in the large arteries to the brain. One of the issues with using this as a screen for stroke, however, is that carotid atherosclerosis probably only covers around 20 to 30 per cent of the causes of stroke; the remainder are due to either emboli (dislodged clots) coming from the heart and large blood vessels, such as the aorta, or disease within the blood vessels in the brain. Thus, although carotid ultrasound screening is very useful, it should not be seen as a foolproof method of screening for stroke.

Mammography has been a suggested routine screening test for women for the past 20 years. It is recommended that women from the age of 50 to 70 have screening mammography performed at least every two years, and those at higher risk more frequently. The place of mammography in women from 40 to 50 and past 70 is still a matter of controversy within the profession. Unfortunately, mammography still misses around 15 per cent of small cancers and although a normal mammogram is reassuring, it does not nullify the need for regular self-examination of the breasts and a yearly examination by a health professional.

Prostate ultrasound is certainly not in the mainstream of preventative screens, but it is now being offered more frequently by some services.

A central part of the executive health screen is the **exercise test**. Many companies have contracts with preventative screening services and a central part of the contract is to perform exercise testing on all the executives of the company. This is done frequently without any questioning of the value of exercise tests. My opinion regarding exercise tests is that they are extremely valuable for middle-age males with typical symptoms of coronary disease, such as chest pain or discomfort during exercise and/or stress. In this situation it is likely that the exercise test will give valuable information. I strongly question, however, the value of exercise testing as a preventative screen for heart disease.

It takes decades for a fatty plaque to form within the wall of an artery and it is only at the last minute at a very late stage that the fatty plaque ruptures through the wall, prompting a clot to form over the ruptured plaque and a subsequent blockage to occur in the artery. Thus, you can have an exercise test the day before your heart attack with a widely open artery; the next day a large fatty plaque that was previously sitting quietly in the wall of the artery can rupture and become a heart attack.

An exercise test cannot predict this. Therefore, as a predictor of future events, the exercise test is of little value. In fact, in this day of modern imaging, I can see no real reason to perform exercise tests without super-added imaging. This can be either in the form of **stress echocardiography** (which is my favoured test) or **stress nuclear testing**, using either an isotope known as thallium or the newer isotope, sestamibi. Both these tests give comparable results in terms of diagnostic ability, the difference being that stress echocardiography is completely non-invasive, not requiring injections of nuclear material, and is about half the price. Also, some of the stress nuclear tests can take up to five hours, whereas stress echocardiography takes only one hour.

Basically, with an exercise test alone, if you group together 100 people with proven coronary artery disease of a significant nature and perform the exercise test you will miss the diagnosis for around 30 out of that 100. Alternatively, if you line up 100 people without coronary artery disease and perform the exercise test, you will over-diagnose potential heart problems in around 30 cases. By adding in imaging you reduce these numbers to 10 false negative diagnoses and 10 false positive diagnoses—an absolute improvement of 20 per cent in both cases.

I have now performed well over 15 000 stress echocardiograms and find them an extremely valuable test. They have a much better predictive value for long-term cardiac events but still nowhere near as accurate as CT scanning of the coronaries. In a recent study, the CT scan could predict in people with scores of greater than 1000 a one-in-four chance of either sudden death or heart attack (if, of course, these people were left untreated). When they compared this group to a comparable set of people with abnormal stress echoes or stress thalliums, their yearly risk was only around 7 per cent.

One of the new, exciting and now available techniques for very early screening of coronary artery disease and future risk for cardiovascular disease is that of **arterial tonometry**. One of the world pioneers of this technique is Professor Michael O'Rourke from Sydney's St Vincent's Hospital. Professor O'Rourke has clearly demonstrated that with the use of this simple, completely non-invasive technique—requiring a blood pressure cuff, an arterial tonometer and a simple software program—the state of health of a person's blood vessels can be determined at a very early age. This simple technique gives an indication of the stiffness of the blood vessels, the function of the endothelium (the lining of the blood vessels), and a few other important parameters. The endothelial cell is the first line of defence to the many poisons that gradually destroy our bodies, and early changes in endothelial cell function can signal future big-league problems in the vascular system.

What about the future?
With the completion of the human genome project, the way of the future will, of course, be genetic screening. Many of these imaging modalities will probably be replaced by the genetic screening clinic. This futuristic, one-stop shop may involve walking in off the street in your early twenties, or possibly even being tested as a newborn. A smear of cells will be taken from the buccal cucosa (the inner lining of the mouth) and all aspects of DNA will be assessed. A percentage ranking for risks for all forms of disease will be determined.

I can see the situation occuring as follows:

John McLachlan is 22 years old. He has smoked since the age of 18 but is thin and plays sport regularly and feels pretty well. His father, however, is 46 years old and has just undergone coronary artery bypass surgery. John's grandfather died aged 53 of a major heart attack. John makes an appointment at the local gene clinic.

His buccal smear is taken and within half an hour he has a comprehensive genetic profie. His risk for atherosclerotic heart disease before the age of 60 is deemed at 95 per cent; his risk for lung cancer is 60 per cent; bowel cancer risk, 10 per cent; prostate cancer, 25 per cent; diabetes, 55 per cent . . . Basically, John is a walking genetic time bomb. The time for John to think about health issues is now, not when he's 40.

With the newer strategies that will be available when these genetic screens are available, many of the above diseases will be prevented completely, and I certainly believe that this will be a reality at some stage in the very near future.

Preventative health clinics

As mentioned above, I believe the preventative health clinic is also the way of the future. For too long we have waited until a disease occurred and then expected a clever member of the medical profession to resurrect our body from the ravages of long-term abuse. To detect and to treat potential problems early must surely be the best method of maintaining health. A preventative health centre, however, should not just be a screening service—it should provide a total service for the individual. A true preventative health service will provide the following levels of care:

- Accurate assessment: Having a true and accurate assessment of all types of common diseases is a vital central role of the preventative health clinic. This includes screening for all types of cardiovascular disease, common cancers (lung and colon; specifically for women: breast, uterine and cervical; and for men: prostate). They should also screen for osteoporosis and the common risk factors for vascular disease and cancer.
- An education program: This will be where the results are discussed, including a comprehensive analysis of the imaging results, the blood tests and the clinical assessment.
- A comprehensive plan: This should be set into place with simple, easy-to-follow instructions. The clients of a preventative health centre should see the centre as their partner in maintaining their health. It is the responsibility of the person to make the behavioural changes, but it is also the responsibility of the clinic to carefully monitor the success of the plan.
- Motivational programs: This will induce the behavioural changes necessary to implement the treatment strategies.
- Follow-up: No program can have success without adequate

follow-up. The strategies set out by the people working at the clinic have to involve not only the right sort of medical advice, but also the appropriate times for follow-up.

No clinic could take the place of a family doctor, but with the increasing time constraints placed on family physicians and those in general practice, there is little time to deal with the primary problem, let alone offer a comprehensive preventative health strategy. Preventative health clinics should work in contact with the person's family doctor to ensure the ongoing good health of the person involved.

Achieve optimum nutrition

Around 10 000 years ago, when we were all hunter–gatherers, and the concept of *quality of life* was just being developed by some primitive marketing executive scratching out some thoughts on the side of his cave somewhere, we all 'just existed'. Human beings at that stage were at the top of the food chain spending most of their time gathering food and avoiding attacks from other tribes and wild animals.

Long before the days of industrial chemists and food technologists, people ate whatever they could get their hands on. Their diet may have included fish skilfully caught with a home-made spear (without expert technical advice from a celebrity hosting a fishing show on television), animals hunted and killed on the day and, of course, wild fruits, nuts, seeds and vegetables gathered from the wild. It is a sad fact, but primitive cardiologists found it very difficult to make a living at that time. First, because there was not much they *could* do, and secondly, because there was not much they *had* to do. Eating was one of life's necessities, not one of the major pleasures it is today.

Over the centuries, different regions of the world developed distinct eating habits based on, obviously, the available food of that region.

Thus, for example, the Inuits traditionally had a very high-fat diet based around sea mammals. They ate fish for protein and whale blubber to regulate their bowel action. (Just between you and me, I can think of much better ways to regulate my bowel action.) Not surprisingly, when the Inuits were exposed to more 'Westernised' foods, such as pasta, bread and, of course, the inevitable sugar, they quickly said, 'Hang the fish and whale blubber—this new stuff is much more tasty!' Out went the traditional diets and in came a diet seen more commonly in Western society.

Interestingly, the Inuits had consumed a high-fat diet that contained a significant amount of good fat, and had little or no atherosclerotic disease. Their main cause of fatal disease by the time they reached the age of 60 or 70, when all human bodies naturally become more frail, was, in fact, cerebral haemorrhage. The reason for this is that they ate too much fish—their blood became too thin. You can't win, can you!

The Westernisation of diets is occurring all around the world. Since the Second World War, the total fat intake of the Japanese diet has increased from around 7 per cent to its current levels in the high 20s (as a percentage of energy intake). This is lower than most developed countries, which have fat contents that make up somewhere between 30 and 40 per cent of their daily energy intake from nutrients. Our tastebuds are not just fixated with fat, though, we also have a love affair with sugar.

Most people cannot and will not accept a diet that is low fat and low sugar. They will accept one or the other, but certainly not both. If you examine the eating trends of any particular area of the world (for those, of course, who have ready access to food), they are either high in fat or high in sugar, or, as in most cases, a combination of both.

The third issue with our diet today is, of course, salt. In cultures where there was little access to salt, as soon as it became more readily available they quickly adopted a much higher salt intake. Salt was largely used as a preservative and when refrigeration became available in most areas the salt intakes dropped to levels we have today.

Subconsciously, the Western way of eating is the preferred way of eating for people. Although cultures do maintain their own traditions, there is a subtle but definite trend towards a 30 to 40 per cent energy intake from fat sources, with around 15 to 20 per cent from protein, and the remainder from varying levels of carbohydrate.

As we have discussed, nutrition is now one of life's pleasures. Unfortunately, most of our food is processed and packaged, and is either too high in fat or sugar, or both. The discipline and time required to cook and prepare meals in these time-poor days, when the alternative is popping a pre-prepared meal into the microwave for a few minutes, presents us with a difficult situation. The average evening meal now takes around five to 10 minutes to consume, usually with the television as the centre of attention. Yet eating still occupies a central place in our social life. You don't say to someone or a group of friends, 'Let's go out for a chat.' You usually go for a meal, a coffee or afternoon tea, usually consuming a piece of cake or some biscuits, promoting each other's coronary disease by these societal rituals.

Over the past 30 to 40 years there has been an explosion of advice about diets and, frankly, most people are confused as to what is the most effective, safe and protective diet they should follow. Unfortunately, the opinions and arguments are as varied and conflicting as any area of life. It is my opinion that it is entirely up to the consumer which advice they follow. In this Information Age, where we no longer kowtow to the opinion of the authorities, we have choice. Unfortunately, that choice does create a degree of anxiety because of the varieties of choice available. It also means that we, as intelligent human beings, can read the evidence and make up our own minds as to what appears to be the most logical.

So we come to a thorny issue: why bother writing yet another book where a large part discusses nutrition? In fact, an even stronger question is: why bother reading yet another book where a large part discusses nutrition? I agree entirely that with so many varying opinions it's becoming more and more difficult to decide who is right and who is wrong. But I must emphasise that the opinions stated by myself throughout this book *are* based on science and *are* based on a global review of literature, and not just a few selected grabs to further my argument. I do believe we have been wrong in our emphasis and that certain aspects of our diet are misplaced, and I hope, in the simplest possible terms (and hopefully in an entertaining and readable way), to present this information and evidence.

Over the past 10 years I personally have taken a strong interest in preventative health and preventative nutrition. I believe I have been able to refine my opinions through careful reading of the majority of literature available on the subject and will present to you what I believe to be an unbiased, scientifically based appraisal of the available evidence. After that—it's entirely up to you to decide what you choose to do about it. I must also state that I have no particular barrow to push. I do not have an affiliation with any particular food, vitamin or nutritional supplement company. I am, however, more than delighted to accept a stipend to promote products that I genuinely believe are of great benefit to humanity.

With such a wonderful and varied amount of food available in modern society, all health experts agree that it is enjoying this variety in moderation that is the pathway to good health. An imbalance has potential for causing harm. My basic message is very simple:

The more synthetic a food or supplement, the more potential for harm. The more natural a food or supplement, the more potential for good.

There are not too many true experts in the field of nutrition who would suggest that a poor diet, obesity and diabetes is particularly good for the body. But I must strongly state that our current nutritional approach of a relatively low-fat, high-carbohydrate diet isn't working. Just walk outside into any major city street and look around. See how many people, including children and young people, are becoming increasingly overweight.

I am reminded of a rather interesting movie called *The Poseidon Adventure*. In this movie, a large ocean liner is turned upside-down by a huge tidal wave. The purser (sounds very much like professor) is supposedly the authority on all matters nautical. He advises all the passengers to sit in the State Room, as help will come. A priest, played by Gene Hackman, says: 'No, this is not right. We must climb up to the bottom of the ship.'

Only five or six people listen to Mr Hackman; the majority choosing to stay with the purser. Within minutes of the minority climbing to safety, a large wave of water sweeps through the State Room killing all the remaining passengers.

Does the bulk of society continue to believe that synthetic foods have been manufactured with love and care by multinational food companies? While we continue to expand at a great rate, we are creating an ever-increasing supply of patients for endocrinologists and cardiologists. When will people start looking to the alternatives?

WEIGHT LOSS

Weight gain is the scourge of modern society—obesity is now an epidemic. It is estimated that 55 per cent of Western society is overweight, with probably around 30 per cent obese. Although there is no doubt that an element of genetics is involved in this situation, the reality is that if any of these overweight people were put in a prison camp and fed a true 'lean cuisine', the weight would drop off at a great rate.

A very depressing statistic is that 97 per cent of those who go on a weight-loss program or specific diet will, three years later, be either the same weight or will have, in fact, gained weight. Although all of the weight-loss programs are effective, their effectiveness is only for the time you maintain the program. I see dieting as analogous to going on a holiday. When you go on a holiday, you come back from a holiday. When you go on a diet, you come back from the diet. In short, diets may take some weight off but it won't take you long to put the weight back on.

Most diets, especially the fad diets, involve a significant loss of water and muscle during the first month. Unless you are on an extremely low-carbohydrate diet, it usually takes somewhere between three and six months to start mobilising fat stores. Therefore, the usual trend on a diet is: one month of alleged success, then a few months of steady weight maintenance, followed by the declaration, 'Blow this, I'm going back to my old eating habits' after seeing no change. Within a further month or two you will have regained all the weight you'd lost. As this weight loss was primarily water and muscle, you now regain fat and become flabbier.

True and sustained weight loss on a permanent basis requires a true and sustained change in your lifestyle habits. If you owned a million-dollar racehorse, would you feed it rubbishy food, ply it with alcohol, give it 20 to 30 cigarettes a day and not exercise it? Of course you wouldn't. We are our own million-dollar racehorses, we are our own greatest assets, and yet we abuse ourselves on a daily basis.

There are two simple principles to losing weight:

- eat less; and
- exercise and move more.

Case study: Tom—Tom is 43 years old. He played grade cricket in his twenties and was also a good swimmer. He married in his late twenties and, following the birth of his first child, succumbed to pressure from his wife to give up his Saturday afternoon sport. Throughout his thirties he rose through the ranks of a prominent financial firm. With increasing seniority came increasing responsibility and increasing time spent at work. He had little time for his family and no time for exercise. His once lean 70-kilogram frame was a rather stocky 105 kilograms by his late thirties.

The healthier eating habits he had during his twenties had also declined. His breakfast consisted of a commercial cereal, a piece of toast and, to help kick-start the day, a strong cup of coffee—with the obligatory two sugars. He had a second cup of strong coffee around mid-morning and often had little time for lunch, so he'd grab a few biscuits about mid-afternoon as his hunger became evident. By the time he arrived home well after 7.30 p.m., he was famished and exhausted. Although his wife tried to prepare good meals, they often ate takeaway food washed down with a few beers. This pattern was repeated week in, week out, with the obligatory dining out with friends on the weekend—Sunday was usually spent recovering from the hangover from Saturday evening. On Monday morning the whole cycle would start again.

Tom's case is far too familiar. In his forties now, he enters the most important decade of his life as far as the direction of his health is concerned. With too much dedication to his work and too much emphasis on creating financial security for his family, Tom has disregarded his greatest asset: himself.

I have no doubt that in the future, effective weight-loss drugs will be available. These may allow us to practise gluttony to our heart's content (pardon the pun), but for the time being, it's your choice. Follow the simple lifestyle principles I am about to expand on and you give yourself the best chance of becoming healthy, and probably a lot happier. Remember, however, the following five rules for weight loss:

1. Weight loss takes time: To lose a significant amount of weight, you need to change your lifestyle permanently. Don't make short-term plans, make long-term goals that will sustain you for the rest of your life.
2. Weight loss needs exercise: Over the age of 35 it is difficult to lose and sustain weight loss by diet alone. Fifty per cent of the weight lost through dieting is fat loss. Weight loss through exercise, however, is 100 per cent fat. In the Mediterranean they have their largest meal at lunchtime and then work during the afternoon, burning off any excess sugar and fat that may cause problems. We tend to have our main meal in the eventing and do no exercise after this.
3. What you eat is important: Remember that breakfast is probably the most important meal of the day and should not be just a piece of toast and a cup of coffee. You may be surprised to learn that a diet involving 'good' fats is more efficient for losing weight than a low-fat, high-carbohydrate diet. Although I'm a great supporter of the Mediterranean diet, I do worry about the amount of pasta it contains. Pasta has a high glycaemic index and therefore, a strong tendency to push out insulin and allow people to gain weight. 'The 19 out 21 rule' states that for 19 meals out of 21 you should stick with your usual eating patterns—the other two meals you can basically eat what you like.
4. Consider your alcohol consumption: One standard glass of wine has around 70 calories, and beer, of course, contains much more than that.

5. Why you eat is important: In Western society we all overeat. When we have too much food on our plate, we tend to consume most of what is there. We are consuming far too much food for our bodies' metabolic needs. Look at why you are really eating what you are eating, and how much your body really needs.

THE GOOD FATS

During the past 30 to 50 years, health professionals in Western society have been obsessed with low-fat eating. In many ways, this obsession has not transferred to the rest of the community, but it has certainly been the catch-cry of health professionals until many started to realise that it wasn't working.

In a strict scientific study, Dr Dean Ornish from California showed that a combined lifestyle program that involved a vegetarian diet with 10 per cent fat, a regulated, five-times-a-week exercise program and regular daily meditation causes a mild reversal in blockages in the coronary arteries and a significant reduction in hard cardiovascular events, such as recurrent heart attack, sudden death and the need for intervention in the form of coronary artery surgery, ballooning or stinting of arteries. Although these results are very impressive, it is difficult to say whether they are due to the very low-fat diet, the exercise program, the meditation or, most likely, a combination of all three.

In the real world, however, you will not find too many people (even those with severe heart disease) who will accept such a rigid lifestyle program, especially the ultra-low-fat diet. Personally, it is my opinion that this type of diet is rather unpalatable and, in fact, the scientific world has clearly shown there are better alternatives.

After the results of the Seven Countries Study performed by Professor Ancel Keys were released, it was clear that the lowest rates of heart disease in the world occurred in Crete, where 40 per cent of their diet was fat. The Japanese also had very low rates of heart disease and, again, a significant proportion of their diet is fish, which is high in fat. The Okinawans (Okinawa is a Japanese island) have the highest rate of people alive and well over the age of 100 in the world. The death rate of the Okinawan people between the age of 60 and 70 is 60 per cent less than the rest of Japan. Their diet contains much more pork and twice the amount of fish compared to the rest of Japan. They have three times less cardiovascular disease, but interestingly consume 40 per cent less calories. The Okinawans and the people of Crete certainly have diets that would not be considered low in fat.

There has never been any study that shows that an isolated reduction in dietary fat or cholesterol will have any benefit at all on increasing longevity in an otherwise healthy person. So, is a low-fat diet a healthy diet? The answer to that is 'possibly', but certainly not 'definitely'.

It is my firm opinion, backed up by many scientific papers, that a truly healthy diet is a diet that is high in 'good' fats. Good fats include pure essential fatty acids with a predominance of Omega-3 fatty acids over pure Omega-6 fatty acids, and mono-unsaturated fatty acids, which include oleic acid and the less common palmitoleic acid. To be more correct, however, rather than calling these substances fats, we should call them lipids.

Lipids do not really dissolve in water, but do so in organic solvents such as chloroform, benzene and ether. Lipids include:

- fatty acids—the most common form being triglycerides, which are three fatty acids linked to a glycerol molecule
- phospholipids—a common one being lecithin
- sterols—the most common being cholesterol.

Lipids that are solid at room temperature are called fats, and lipids that are liquid at room temperature are called oils.

The different types of fatty acids include:

- saturated fat—especially animal fats and milk products, but other substances, such as coconuts, are also high in saturated fats
- mono-unsaturated fats—olive oil, canola oil, avocado, nuts
- polyunsaturated fats—divided into Omega-3s (fish and plant-derived) or Omega-6s (usually from vegetable oils)
- trans fatty acids—the worst type of fatty acid, which is the synthetic form of unsaturated fats.

LOW FAT VERSUS GOOD FAT

The Lyon Diet Heart Study discussed in the 'Chronic nutritional poisoning' chapter, compared a diet high in mono-unsaturated fats and essential fatty acids (a Mediterranean diet) with a standard low-fat diet. It demonstrated a significant 75 per cent reduction in subsequent heart attack, stroke and sudden death for those on the standard Mediterranean diet using liberal amounts of mono-unsaturated and Omega-3 fatty acids. If you take a standard cholesterol-lowering pill, known as a statin, there is only around a 20 to 30 per cent reduction in heart attack, stroke and cardiac-related death. The low-fat diet was obviously the wrong diet for this group.

In another study, performed in India, 400 people who survived a heart attack were given either a standard low-fat diet or a diet high in nuts, legumes and essential oils but no meat. After six weeks there was a 36 per cent reduction in all cardiac events for those on the diet high in nuts, etc. Again, the low-fat diet didn't work.

The best explanation for this comes from a study performed on rats in South Australia. The rats were divided into three groups. Each rat had the main artery in their heart tied, thus inducing a major heart attack. The first group was given a diet similar to the highly processed diet seen in our society. The second group was given a standard diet with around 25 to 30 per cent fat. The third group was given a diet low in bad fats but high in mono-unsaturated and Omega-3 fatty acids. All of the rats in the first group died suddenly. Half of the rats in the second group died suddenly. None of the rats in the third group died suddenly.

The reason for this is quite clear. Your heart is at its most irritable when you're having a heart attack. The worst thing you can give an irritated heart is a poison that irritates it, such as bad fat. But to take the fat away altogether leaves the heart unprotected. To add in good fats, which stabilise cardiac membranes and stop the heart from being irritable, gives the greatest benefit. Thus the benefit with the rats, the Indians and the French.

Another area where the low-fat diet advocates are not thinking clearly is in regards to the cell membrane, which is so vital in general nutrition. It is composed of 75 per cent fat. Without a constant supply of the good fats and/or an excessive supply of the bad fats in the form of trans fatty acids, the membrane soon gets disrupted and becomes hard and impermeable. Nutrients cannot then make their way into the cell because the delivery system (the membrane) isn't doing its job. The other concern I have is that a sudden and acute change in the cholesterol and fat content of membranes can also alter normal membrane function. But in certain circumstances, such as many forms of cardiovascular disease, excessive amounts of cholesterol and fats in the bloodstream do cause harm and need to be treated. Unfortunately, however, many people who are not getting adequate assessments of their true risk for vascular disease are given cholesterol-lowering agents or are told to follow a low-fat regimen purely on the basis of a blood cholesterol estimation.

If you have definite evidence for vascular disease (as seen on CT scanning of the coronary arteries) or a very strong family history of premature heart disease, then it is highly likely your vascular disease will cause you bother. Therefore, it is very justified in this situation to aggressively manage cholesterol levels with a combination of choles-terol-lowering diet and exercise or with statin drugs. But we now have the bizarre situation where some US cardiologists recommend patients who have totally normal cholesterol levels and no real risk for heart disease take statin agents on a *preventative* basis.

Essential fatty acids

'Essential' basically means that it is vital we swallow the stuff. All nutri-tion experts are happy to call the Omega-3 and Omega-6 fatty acids 'essential fatty acids'. So what are these Omega-3 and Omega-6 fatty acids? Why are they essential? And how much do we really need?

The Omega-3 and Omega-6 fatty acids are the polyunsaturated fats. Saturated fat is a fat that lacks double carbon bonds and an unsaturated fat is a fat that has double carbon bonds in its chain. These subtle differences between chemicals have an enormous difference on how they work in the body.

The essential fatty acids have five main functions:

1. to ensure cell membrane functions correctly;
2. to maintain balance within the body functions through the eicosanoid compound;
3. to aid normal functioning of the brain and retina;
4. to reduce cholestereol and aid fat metabolism; and
5. to boost the immune system.

1. CELL MEMBRANES

Seventy five per cent of every cell membrane is made of fat and of this fat, around 30 per cent is essential fatty acids. The membrane is the first port of call of nutrients, so it is a vital part of the cell. As I have already stated, if your membrane isn't working properly, your cell cannot work properly. Without the right balance of essential fatty acids in your diet your cells soon become defective and cannot function properly. Ridding your body of trans fatty acids and replacing these with essential fatty acids restores normal cellular function. Trans fatty acids harden the membrane and make it impermeable to nutrients; whereas the essential fatty acids make the membrane more fluid, allowing essential nutrients to cross the membrane into the cell easily so the cells can perform their normal function.

2. EICOSANOIDS

Essential fatty acids are the major component of a group of compounds known as eicosanoids. Eicosanoids maintain the local balance in and around the cells. Look at it this way: life is really a balance between good and bad, short and tall, smart and no-so-smart—an analogy that can be applied to all of the functions of the body. I have mentioned our fear–fight–flight system and the opposing relaxation system. For the body to maintain balance, it has to be able to choose at any particular time which part of the spectrum in all aspects of metabolism and life it needs to be. If everything is functioning smoothly, the body can maintain its system somewhere in the middle in what we call 'homeostasis'. If, however, the body is acutely stressed, it needs to have mechanisms to cope with this stress. The eicosanoids perform many of the local functions to maintain this balance. For example, the contraction or relaxation of muscles, and the clotting or free flowing of blood. You will be well aware of the 'Economy Syndrome' regarding plane travel. This is not just simple bad luck. It is caused by people who have more of a tendency to clotting than a tendency to bleeding. There are many genetic and acquired clotting defects that can predispose an affected person to form clots, especially in the veins in their legs and pelvis. These clots dislodge and can get stuck in the lungs, causing the so-called 'Economy Syndrome'. Medically, this is known as 'deep vein thrombosis' and subsequent 'pulmonary embolus'. In someone with a normal heart it is impossible for the clot to travel beyond the lung, but if it is a large clot it can actually block completely the inflow into the lung and, in some cases, cause death.

If a person has a tendency towards clotting and they sit cramped in a place for a number of hours, this is a common precipitant to a clot forming. When they start moving their legs, the movement dislodges the clot that has formed and the clot, unfortunately, can often end up in the lungs. Therefore, Economy Syndrome is really not caused by sitting in the economy section of a plane but is, in fact, caused by people who have a genetic predisposition to clotting formation being in a situation where they are immobilised for a period of time. This is especially so if their legs are bent in a cramped position. To sue an airline for this condition is absolutely ridiculous and lacks any medical common sense. It is an unfortunate occurrence which may have happened if the person, who is genetically predisposed, lies in a hospital bed for a week, takes a prolonged car trip, or has a plaster cast on their leg.

What has all this got to do with eicosanoids? Well, the balance between Omega-3 and Omega-6 fatty acids in your body will affect the eicosanoids produced.

The Omega-6 fatty acids are the most commonly consumed fatty acids; usually in a ratio of about 10:1 (Omega-6 to Omega-3). The average person requires around 1 per cent of their daily energy intake in the form of Omega-6 fatty acids, which is usually around 2 to 4 grams per day. The usual Western diet contains much less Omega-3 fatty acids. Conservative nutritionists suggest anywhere between 0.2 to 0.5 grams of Omega-3 should be consumed per day but in my opinion this causes an imbalance in eicosanoid production. If we have too much Omega-6 fatty acids we consume too much linoleic acid, which is the main Omega-6 fatty acid, and generate too much arachidonic acid.

Why am I boring you with all this science? Because it is important to know that arachidonic acid creates a very important prostaglandin (which is a by-product of eicosanoids) known as thromboxane A-2. This particular prostaglandin has two rather nasty actions:

- It makes those sticky little cells in your bloodstream known as 'platelets' even stickier.
- It constricts arteries.

On the other hand, the Omega-3 essential fatty acids generate a chemical known as alpha-linolenic acid, which is the plant-based form of Omega-3; or, if you consume Omega-3s from marine sources, they generate either eicosapentaenoic acid (EPA) or docosahexaenoic acid (DHA). When you increase the amount of Omega-3 in your diet, these substances create a different prostaglandin known as prostacyclin. This has the opposite effects to thromboxane A-2. Prostacyclin is made in the endothelial cell lining of blood vessels and stops the platelets from being sticky (therefore thinning the blood) and dilates blood vessels, therefore improving the blood flow.

It is important to get a balance between these substances not to rush out and have 30 to 40 per cent of your energy intake in Omega-3 fatty acids, as your blood will become too thin and your blood vessels too prone to breaking down through excessive blood flow. Like everything I say, it is important to achieve a balance.

I must state, however, that I believe that we are not achieving that balance with our current dietary methods. It is vital we have a certain degree of Omega-6 polyunsaturated fats but I believe we should be markedly increasing our Omega-3 polyunsaturated fats so that the ratio is no longer 10:1, but closer to 3:1.

3. THE BRAIN AND THE RETINA

The brain and the retina are particular sensitive structures that require a regular amount of essential fatty acids for normal functioning. The blood-brain barrier is an important barrier used to protect the brain from internal toxins. It is basically a fat-soluble region that requires a significant amount of essential fatty acids for normal functioning.

4. CHOLESTEROL AND FAT METABOLISM

One of the major factors in generation of a high cholesterol level is the fatty acid composition of the bloodstream. Diets high in trans fatty acids, and to a lesser extent saturated fat, generate high levels of LDL cholesterol. Diets high in polyunsaturated fats, or mono-unsaturated fats, tend to drop the LDL cholesterol levels. One of the recommendations has been to increase polyunsaturated fats in the diet and also to increase carbohydrate concentration. Unfortunately, this combination leads to a lower total cholesterol, but also a lower HDL cholesterol and a high triglyceride concentration. If the essential fatty acids are increased in the bloodstream, especially with an increased ratio of Omega-3 to Omega-6 fatty acids along with a decrease in processed carbohydrates, the LDL (or bad cholesterol) will fall, but the HDL will either remain stable or, in some cases, increase. One of the most important points to note is that essential fatty acids will very rapidly be oxidised if there are not adequate antioxidant vitamins to protect them. It is, therefore, recommended that in diets high in essential fatty acids, additional Vitamin E is consumed—which I believe should be done anyhow.

5. THE IMMUNE SYSTEM

The eicosanoids, as I have mentioned, are a vital part of essential fatty acid metabolism. They are also very important controlling chemicals for immune function. Excessive amounts of arachidonic acid from the Omega-6 fatty acids tend to be pro-inflammatory. This is one of the proposed mechanisms for the increase of arthritis and asthma in our society, whereas increasing the Omega-3 essential fatty acids has been shown to have an anti-inflammatory action. High doses of Omega-3 supplements are now being used in the treatment of numerous arthritic conditions.

Any chronic inflammatory condition may be affected by the essential fatty acids, especially if the balance of these is upset or we are not achieving an adequate amount in our diet. Chronic inflammation is said to play a major role in the generation of heart disease. A component of white cells known as macrophages are felt to be part of the earliest lesions of atherosclerosis (the fatty plaque). When a macrophage ingests the free radical–affected oxidised LDL cholesterol, the inflammatory macrophage becomes a 'foam' cell. These foam cells coalesce to become a progressively increasing fatty plaque. Other components of the white cell brigade, when stimulated by an inflammatory response, can then erode the lining of the plaques contributing to plaque rupture, which is the major event that occurs during a heart attack. Therefore, achieving the right balance of essential fatty acids is an important step in reducing the risk for the development of atherosclerosis in the first place, and the subsequent complication of a ruptured fatty plaque leading to the major consequences of atherosclerosis—heart attack, stroke and sudden cardiac death.

Common sources of essential fatty acids

One of the important points to make regarding the intake of fats is that there is usually a mix of different fats in the one food. For example, meat does not just contain saturated fat, there is also a proportion of mono-unsaturated fats as well. Olive oil, which is known as the major rich source of mono-unsaturated fats (around 77 per cent) is 14 per cent saturated fat. Coconut oil, on the other hand, is only 6 per cent mono-unsaturated fat and around 92 per cent saturated fat. It is more important, however, to look at the major fat within the food and to look at the effects of taking this whole food.

As mentioned earlier, the Seven Countries Study showed that the Japanese have a low rate of heart disease due to their low intake of saturated fat—of the 25 per cent total fat intake, only 7 per cent was from saturated fat. The people of Crete had an even lower rate of heart disease than the Japanese. While 40 per cent of their diet was in fat, most was from the consumption of olive oil.

FISH

The most common source of essential fatty acids is from fish, especially fatty fish such as salmon, tuna or sardines. The regular consumption of two to three fish meals each week has been shown in varying studies to reduce the risk for a heart attack by around 30 per cent. When the studies are viewed very carefully, this is almost entirely due to a reduction in sudden cardiac death. The reason is felt to be due to the Omega-3 fatty acids having a stabilising effect on cell membranes, especially the electrical system in the heart. There is also, of course, the element of the anti-inflammatory component, which stops the rupturing of plaques. It is the large plaques that rupture in the major arteries tending to cause the severe electrical disturbance that leads to a cardiac arrest and subsequent cardiac death.

One trial, known as the DART study (Diet and Reinfarction Trial), showed a 32 per cent reduction in coronary heart disease mortality and a 29 per cent reduction in all-cause mortality with the consumption of oily fish on at least two occasions per week. Another study, known as the Western Electric Trial from Chicago, showed the same reduction in cardiac death—even in people not consuming particularly oily fish. Regardless, there is no doubt that the regular consumption of fish on a weekly basis, on at least two occasions, can have a significant and profound effect on reducing your risk for cardiovascular disease and death.

NUTS

For many years, nuts have been maligned as a source of fat that can contribute to a premature demise. Over the past 10 years, however, there have been five separate studies demonstrating that the consumption of natural nuts in low doses leads to around a 50 per cent reduction in cardiac disease when people are studied over a long period of time. The most notable of these studies was the Adventists' Health Study, which studied 36 000 people from California. When the researchers looked at their diet over 12 years, there was a clear independent benefit from nut consumption.

Of course, I'm not referring to the sort of nuts roasted in vegetable oil and salted, I mean natural nuts. Not only do these nuts contain wonderful proteins, they are also rich in essential fatty acids with a good balance of Omega-3 and Omega-6, and also the other good form of fat, mono-unsaturated fat. I believe the three nuts that achieve the best long-term results are walnuts, almonds and macadamias. All nuts, however, except for maybe cashews (which do have a significant amount of saturated fat), are good for you in low doses. I suggest that 10 to 15 nuts a day is the right dose.

EGGS
The much maligned eggs are a wonderful source of essential fatty acids. In each egg there is around 5 grams of fat, of which 3 grams are from mono-unsaturated fat and polyunsaturated fat. The remainder is a combination of saturated fat and cholesterol. With a diet low in trans fatty acids, I do not believe the cholesterol content of an egg is particularly important and will not have huge impact on serum cholesterol level.

A few years back, the *New England Journal of Medicine* reported the case of one man who consumed 12 eggs each day and had a totally normal serum cholesterol level. I believe the cholesterol in eggs will only cause a problem if it is associated with other food sources that contain trans fatty acids, such as cakes, biscuits, french toast, pancakes and cookies. The trans fatty acids from sources other than the egg are of much more concern than the egg itself.

Eggs are also a wonderful source of protein and, although the nutritionists tell us we should only be having two eggs each week, I believe one egg a day is quite healthy. These days, eggs can also be enriched with Omega-3 fatty acids, which makes them even better for you.

OILS
Canola oil has a higher ratio of Omega-3 to Omega-6 than soy-bean oil, although both are good sources. There has been much misinformation circulating regarding canola oil. Canola oil was initially developed through traditional plant breeding methods and not through genetic engineering or irradiation. It has been shown in recent studies to be of great benefit.

There is also much misinformation disseminated regarding margarine. I am concerned about the use of a sunflower oil– or safflower oil–based margarine because of the trans fatty acid content. The trans fatty acid content of margarines, however, even from the Omega-6 polyunsaturated forms, have been markedly reduced. The newer margarines with a canola oil and/or olive oil base are an excellent source of essential fatty acids.

The Lyon Diet Heart Study (discussed previously) showed a spectacular benefit in the group who ate the Mediterranean-style diet, enriched with alpha linolenic acid from a canola oil-based margarine. Although I am not attributing all of the benefits seen in the study to alpha linolenic acid (a wonderful essential fatty acid source), I do believe this was an important component of the diet and all sources of essential fatty acids should be encouraged as part of our normal day-to-day eating habits.

LSA

LSA is an unprocessed grain mix made from pure linseed, sunflower seeds and almonds. It is a wonderful source of essential fatty acids and I would strongly encourage you to purchase a packet of LSA from either your health food store or supermarket and eat this on a daily basis.

DR WALKER'S SUPER-CHARGED BREAKFAST

A wonderful way to start the day is with a healthy breakfast. I encourage you to try the following breakfast on a regular basis:

- 10 to 15 natural nuts (preferably walnuts, almonds and macadamias).
- 1 to 2 dessertspoons of LSA.
- 1 generous dessertspoon of unprocessed bran.
- a combination of blueberries, strawberries and banana.
- low-fat milk.

This essential fatty acid 'hit' will give you enormous energy first thing in the morning and reduce your craving for processed carbohydrates.

For those of you either allergic or unable to tolerate seafood, using flaxseed or linseed oil is an excellent source of Omega-3 fatty acids. It is important to remember, however, that flaxseeds rapidly become rancid, so they should be used as fresh as possible. Don't forget to use a Vitamin E supplement when you are having a diet high in essential fatty acids.

Essential fatty acid supplements

The most common and cheapest form of essential fatty acid supplements is fish oil capsules. These usually come in a dose of around 1000 milligrams per capsule. I suggest, as a maintenance dose, either one to two capsules a day. For people with chronic inflammatory states, such as rheumatoid arthritis, doses of two twice a day are suggested. Cholesterol abnormalities are usually only reduced in much higher doses— somewhere between the 3–9 gram range. The problem with this is that the person ingesting these capsules at that dose has a persistent 'fishy' taste in their mouth and their breath can actually smell like fish. At much lower doses, this does not occur.

A recent study in Italy of 11 000 people after a heart attack showed that those who took one capsule of fish oil per day had a small, but significant, reduction in further cardiac events, such as heart attack and sudden cardiac death.

Plant-based Omega-3 supplements usually contain around 0.5 grams of Omega-3 and 0.2 grams of Omega-6 fatty acids per capsule. I personally believe that it is a good idea to supplement with an essential fatty acid at this dose, taking two capsules per day.

Common sources of mono-unsaturated fats

Mono-unsaturated fatty acids have been shown to lower total cholesterol levels, but also to have either a neutral or beneficial effect on HDL or 'good' cholesterol levels. They have also been shown to decrease or have no effect on triglycerides.

OLIVE OIL

There is increasing evidence that diets that include a significant amount of olive oil are of great benefit. The oil used in the Mediterranean diet is usually extra-virgin olive oil, which is the first pressing of the olives. Not only is this high in mono-unsaturated fats, but it is also a plentiful source of antioxidants in the form of polyphenols. Studies from Greece have also shown lower rates of breast cancer in those women who regularly consume olive oil.

There has been much conjecture regarding the loss of nutrients with cooking. Professor David Roberts from the University of Newcastle, New South Wales, performed a study where he reheated olive oil 40 times. It did not lose much of its nutrient value with extra reheating.

The benefits of olive oil are undeniable. I am not suggesting, however, you should swim in it, but use a small amount for cooking, on your salads and, if you wish, as an alternative to margarine or butter. The evidence is rather strong that it will help—and let's not forget the superb taste!

CANOLA OIL

Although olive oil gets most of the press regarding its qualities as an oil, its poorer cousin canola oil still has many benefits. It is around 60 per cent mono-unsaturated fat and has the added benefit of being at least 10 per cent Omega-3 polyunsaturated fat. Probably in the setting of people with established heart disease, there is even more benefit in using canola oil rather than olive oil because of the protective effects of the Omega-3 against sudden cardiac death. That's why I am impressed with the combination of canola and olive oils in some of the latest margarines. Although these margarines tend to highlight the fact they are high in olive oil, in reality, the mix is 30 per cent olive oil and 70 per cent canola oil. Similar margarines were used in the Lyon Diet Heart Study with such a profound benefit.

AVOCADO

There has been concern expressed about the use of avocado by some conservative nutritionists. My friend and colleague Dr David Colquhoun, who is a clinical professor of cardiology in Queensland, performed a study where he fed people one half to one avocado per day for a month. Their cholesterols dropped and they lost weight. There was also no change in the HDL (good cholesterol level) in those using the avocados. When the same group of people were switched to a high-carbohydrate diet, it had minimal effect on their total cholesterol but a drop in HDL of around 13 per cent was noted.

Avocados are also a rich source of folic acid. There is around 70 micrograms of folic acid (approximately one-fifth of my recommended daily dose) in a full avocado. Avocados contain significant amounts of potassium as well, and lesser amounts of phosphorus and magnesium. Potassium has been shown to have a significant effect on lowering blood pressure. There are also small amounts of Vitamin C and Vitamin E in avocados.

Avocados contain a significant amount of the same type of cholesterol-lowering substances that are found in the new cholesterol-lowering margarines. Therefore, they make an excellent food package. Not only do they drop cholesterol and assist in weight loss, but they are also a rich source of minerals and vitamins (including folic acid), and are completely natural.

NUTS

One of the problems with suggesting nuts are beneficial is that it makes people believe they have open slather on any form of nuts available. These include the nuts that have been roasted, salted or had some sort of treatment, usually with hydrogenated vegetable oils, creating trans fatty acids. It is the trans fatty acids that have caused all the issues with nuts and not the nuts themselves.

Walnuts and almonds, in particular, are a rich source of essential fatty acids and also contain a significant amount of mono-unsaturated fat. Macadamia nuts have their own special properties, which make them very attractive from a health viewpoint. The common form of mono-unsaturated fat is oleic acid. Macadamia nuts also have palmitoleic acid, which appears to have an even better effect on reducing blood viscosity (keeping the blood flowing) compared with normal oleic acid. My attitude is, rather than just concentrate on either macadamias, walnuts or almonds, have them all together in a mixture every day.

How much good fat do we need?

The argument about how much we really need every day comes back to the same argument as with vitamins. Conservative nutritionists will tell us we only need the recommended daily allowance and anything above that dose is excreted in the urine—the old 'expensive urine', patronising argument. Conservative nutritionists insist also that we only need around 1 or 2 per cent of our total energy intake from essential fatty acids. If your diet is around 2500 kilocalories, you will get all the fatty acids you need in about one tablespoon of some form of vegetable oil. This can be in the form of margarine, mayonnaise, salad dressings, wholegrains or vegetables. No-one disagrees that a deficiency of essential fatty acids below this level can lead to skin problems, diarrhoea and a tendency to other infections. A person will quickly become anaemic and, especially around the time of surgery when people often do not achieve proper nutrition, there will be defective wound healing.

Rather than talking in percentage of energy or grams (which is basically just confusing and very difficult for those of us on the street who don't have the sophisticated measuring devices to sort them out), I will make more straightforward suggestions:

Essential fatty acids

Fish	2 to 3 fish meals per week—preferably fatty fish, such as salmon, tuna and sardines
Fish oil capsules	1000 milligrams—one capsule twice daily
LSA	1 to 2 large dessertspoons per day
Nuts	10 to 15 nuts per day—preferably walnuts, almonds and macadamias

An optional, but recommended, essential fatty acid supplement (apart from fish oil capsules, which are high in alpha linolenic acid compared with linoleic acid) should contain 0.5 grams of alpha linolenic acid per capsule and around 0.2 grams of linoleic acid per capsule.

Mono-unsaturated fats	
Extra-virgin olive oil or canola oil	Use in cooking (extra-virgin olive oil can be reheated); make your own salad dressing using extra-virgin olive oil and balsamic vinegar; use extra-virgin olive oil as a dip for wholegrain bread
Avocado	Half to one avocado per day
Nuts	10 to 15 per day—preferably walnuts, almonds and macadamias

ANTIOXIDANTS

Antioxidants have been one of the nutritional buzzwords thrown around over the past 10 years. We are constantly being told of the benefits of these magical substances and that we should be consuming significant amounts. We have also been given much misinformation from both sides of the nutritional world. The conservative nutritionists tell us we get all the antioxidants we need from our food, while the makers of natural and synthetic vitamins tell us we must use supplements for good health. To understand antioxidants you must understand a little bit of science. First, let me make some analogies using something natural and something less natural.

If you slice an apple through and leave it exposed to air for even a relatively short time, it will start to go brown on the exposed surface. The reason is that when the apple's inner surface is exposed to oxygen there is a reaction known as oxidation, which quickly changes all of the wonderful nutritional benefits within the apple. If you take your car to the beach and leave it there for a few months, you'll find the salt air has rusted the metal of your car. This is also an oxidation process, similiar to what's happening with the apple.

It is also what occurs in the body. When natural processes or unnatural processes occur within the body, oxygen and energy is required to effect these processes, and the cells and the chemicals within the cells become oxidised. Usually, this is not a good thing, and the body has mechanisms to restore the cell or the chemical reaction back to what is known as the 'reduced' state. Human cells generally function in a reduced state. When we think of something being reduced, we think of it losing some value, but in fact, in this particular situation it is better and more efficient for the body to be in a reduced state for most of its chemical reactions to take place.

When oxygen reacts with our energy fuels, such as glucose or free fatty acids, it creates a substance known as ATP in the mitochondria of cells. This ATP is the major energy source that drives almost all of the cellular reactions within the body. When the cell is depleted of ATP it becomes fatigued; when we're depleted of ATP because of this we are also fatigued.

Once the body becomes overloaded with toxins from any source, these toxins have to be dealt with within the cell. The oxygen and other fuel sources have to generate energy to deal with these toxins and very quickly, free radicals are formed. Free radicals are the by-products of these reactions. They are basically unstable chemicals that have lost an electron during the oxidation process. This loss of an electron makes them unstable. They can only gain stability by taking an electron from somewhere, so these nasty little critters then decide to rip an electron from your blood vessels, your LDL cholesterol, your immune system or other cells and also, at times, your DNA. They then go on their merry way, being quite stable with the electron restored. Now, however, your normal cellular functions have been completely screwed up because *they* are unstable and lack these electrons. Thus, the long process of heart disease and cancer begins.

Recent evidence has shown that cardiovascular and cancer rates in people living in cities (especially heavily polluted cities) are about 30 per cent higher than in countryfolk. All of these different exposures, whether they be chemical or some form of radiation, have a final common pathway, which is the generation of free radicals.

Causes of free radicals

So what are the sources of free radicals in our environment? I would like to divide these into the five obvious causes:

1. food
2. exercise
3. stress
4. cigarette smoke
5. pollution

and the five less obvious causes:

1. radiation
2. chemicals
3. pesticides, herbicides, insecticides . . .
4. steroids, antibiotics and genetically modified foods
5. microbes.

FOOD
I will discuss later the different components of food and the different abilities of different types of food to cause and generate free radicals. For now, suffice to say, most of us are overfed and the more food we eat, the more we are stressing our biological systems and oxidising our natural chemicals.

EXERCISE
There is no doubt that the human body is designed for movement. This design, however, is certainly centred around the principles of balance. This balance, known as homeostasis, can adjust for stress, but not too much. Thus, if you avoid regular exercise you will become obese, and that puts a stress on your body.

Alternatively, we hear often of the fit person in their forties and fifties who drops dead while out jogging. In his book *The Antioxidant Revolution*, Dr Ken Cooper from the Cooper Clinic in Dallas basically admits he was wrong in his earlier books on aerobics. It takes a great man and a great thinker to realise the dogma being preached for many years is not always correct. Dr Cooper now admits that high-impact exercise is probably not particularly good for the body.

Research over the past 10 years has clearly shown that high-performance athletes, or people who excessively exercise for any reason, generate significant amounts of free radicals. This is why exercise physiologists and biochemists involved in sports nutrition developed very strong and rigid antioxidant programs for their athletes. Almost all high-performance athletes supplement these days with antioxidants because the demands of their rigorous exercise–training regimen are such that their bodies without compensatory doses of antioxidant vitamins quickly de-compensate due to the free radicals. This is why you often hear of many athletes developing recurrent viruses.

In a fit young person it is unlikely these extra free radicals will cause acute cardiovascular disease or cancer but, certainly, the free radicals will attack the immune system rendering the white cells less efficient and, therefore, predisposing a person to recurrent infections such as colds and flu.

STRESS
In the section on stress I define stress as 'a great pressure or strain'. This strain on the body can come from any form of either physical, mental or emotional stress. I have already discussed the physical stress of exercise, but it can also be the physical stress of trauma to the body. Significant injury to any part of the body can damage the cells. The damaged products of cells generate free radicals in the same way that damaged muscles from excessive exercise do.

Therefore, when any person's body is weakened by a major accident or injury, it is important to compensate by increasing the antioxidant dose for the recovery.

Almost all of us have experienced a viral illness when we are run-down. If we are too busy at work or are undergoing some significant emotional trauma, our bodies release two basic stress hormones: adrenaline and cortisone. Both of these chemicals generate an increased metabolic rate and require more ATP. The more ATP used, the more free radicals are produced. Therefore, there is a clear physiological reaction to stress which has a damaging physical component through the generation of free radicals.

CIGARETTE SMOKE
Cigarette smoking is an excellent way of guaranteeing a constant supply of free radicals bombarding your body.

POLLUTION

In polluted environments, we are constantly being attacked by thousands of different types of vicious poisons. The real cancer of our earth is over-population. Overpopulation induces overuse of resources, which generates a whole host of waste products that contain any number of chemical poisons that destroy our body. Unfortunately in life there is no 'free lunch': if you choose to live in a city and enjoy the benefits of that city you have to tolerate a degree of pollution.

A radical solution I would propose (which will ensure I will never go into politics and certainly never be elected) is to have a toll on all major roads in all major cities. All the revenue collected from these tolls should then be ploughed into efficient, non-polluting forms of public transport. Unfortunately, we have come to the point of believing that driving our own car is our birthright, and hang the effect we are having on the environment.

RADIATION

We derive radiation from many sources. These days every man and his dog sits in front of a computer for a few hours every day and there is certainly a degree of background radiation coming off computers. Sitting too close to the television screen will do the same thing. All manner of electronics can generate a degree of radiation. The two sources in particular I'd like to mention are the microwave and mobile telephones. I would send out a plea to anyone owning a microwave oven (which is most of us) not to stand anywhere near the microwave when you are cooking something. Who knows exactly what it's doing, but let's bring in some common sense regarding this.

What is the story with mobile phones? First, let me say I cannot be confident either way whether mobile phones are safe or not safe. As a paranoid cardiologist I still have a radiation protection shield on my mobile phone, which I'm told by the manufacturers reduces the radiation from the phone by about 99 per cent. Multinational phone companies are always assuring us that there is absolutely nothing wrong with using mobile phones. But please don't forget that back in the '50s and '60s the cigarette companies reassured us there was absolutely nothing wrong with smoking cigarettes. I believe mobile phones are a necessity in our modern age, but my advice is firstly use some form of radiation shield, and secondly, use the phone as little as possible. (Of course, as you can probably guess, I'm not sponsored by a major telecommunications company.)

CHEMICALS

All of the additives, colourings and preservatives or the stuff we use to wash our hair, clean our bodies, paint our faces or make our bodies smell nice—not to mention all of the chemicals we clean surfaces with and clean the cutlery we eat with—deliver micro doses of harmful chemicals into our bodies every day. These chemicals may be of absolutely no consequence and are in such small doses that our bodies' natural systems deal with them immediately and without concern. This may be the scenario—or it may not. No-one has really explained this to my satisfaction as yet and I'm not sure that we will ever really know.

We hear of the occasional person who was allegedly allergic to the twentieth and probably now the twenty-first century. These people's lives appear to be a misery. They get all sorts of skin reactions, respiratory tract infections and gastrointestinal problems when they are exposed to any form of synthetic chemicals. Some doctors think it is a purely psychological reaction and others take it very seriously.

PESTICIDES, HERBICIDES, INSECTICIDES . . .
And any other 'icide' you'd like to mention

The overpopulation of our world means our resources are being stretched to the limit. We therefore have to ensure a constant supply of raw materials for our food supply. No-one, however, explained this to the insect world—they actually quite enjoy feasting on whatever fruit and vegetables are available in their area. Unfortunately, these insects do not pay the farmer a particularly good price for the consumption of the farmer's products, therefore, the farmer tends to use a few tricks of his own to stop the little nuisances attacking his crop. Most crops are sprayed with some form of pesticide which, again, *may* be causing us absolutely no bother whatsoever. I still always wonder and ask the question, 'What is a *safe* level of poison?'

STEROIDS, ANTIBIOTICS AND GENETICALLY MODIFIED FOOD

If you believe the food industry, nothing 'in particular' is added to food. If you believe the conspiracy theorists every 'nasty' possible is thrown into our food supply purely to fill the pockets of those greedy multinationals. Are chickens fed steroids to bulk up their muscles to make them more attractive for sale? How many antibiotics are given to cattle and poultry? To what degree is our food genetically modified?

The next question is: if any of these processes are occurring in our animals and plants, do they have an affect on our bodies?

I must say, no-one has presented to me any convincing evidence either way that really and adequately answers any of these questions. In the same way that we really do not know what the micro-doses of chemicals we are being exposed to every day are doing to our bodies, we also don't know *if* anything is being done to our animals or plants apart from the natural process of growth, if it is being done, what it's doing to us.

You can't live in a bubble and separate yourself away from society. Society has now created a method of acquiring, packaging and distributing food that most of us have come to accept. Whether we like it or not, this is the system that has been created, and short of breeding your own animals and growing your own food in your own environment, my only suggestion along these lines is to make the healthiest choice possible with the most educated advice.

I still eat meat and I still eat poultry. I still eat fish despite people saying that many fish supplies now have excessive levels of poison, such as mercury, which makes the fish a less than nutritious choice. I still eat fruit and vegetables despite the fact that there is a suggestion that they are genetically modified to some extent. And I cetainly take in a significant amount of antioxidant supplements to try to neutralise any possible damaging effects from these subtle micropoisons.

MICROBES

Our body is made up of around 100 trillion cells, in 90 trillion of which there are probably different types of microbes living on our skin and in our gastrointestinal tracts and the upper respiratory tract. Normally, we live in wonderful, peaceful harmony with these bacteria. With the increasing use of antibiotics, however, and the increasing emergence of super bacteria and weird new viruses that can create all manner of havoc within our bodies, we are not only battling a whole group of hidden (and not so hidden) chemicals, but we now face a new wave of bacterial viruses and other parasites.

From the moment you wake up in the morning to the moment you wake up the next day, there is some sort of chemical doing its stuff to your body and your body's intricate metabolic systems. This chemical load on the body's systems generates far too many of these free radicals for us to handle with our natural antioxidant system. There are, therefore, only two things we can do about this free-radical attack on our body.

First, attempt to reduce exposure to free radicals—and I must say, in Western society, it is rather difficult to avoid many of these chemicals. Second, attempt to neutralise these free radicals with antioxidants.

Antioxidants contain a whole host of extra electrons they can donate to these selfish little free radicals and send them on their merry way. For example, Vitamin E, being a fat-soluble vitamin, attaches itself to the outer coating of LDL (the bad cholesterol). When the free radicals come along, they are confronted by Vitamin E, which says, 'No, don't take the LDL electrons, take mine', thus rendering the free radical harmless and protecting the LDL. But some doctors do not believe antioxidants work.

One of the wonderful things about our world is 'difference'. We are all different, we all have different views, and we are all basically different people. Each person is their own little microcosm living within their own world and interacting with the microcosms of millions of other people. In any one community you will have a differing number of views, and this is certainly no different from the world of science.

Within the medical scientific community there is a strong element that pushes the line that you get all of the antioxidants you need from your diet—a diet rich in fruits and vegetables, tea and extra-virgin olive oil—and that vitamins don't work. On the other hand, there is a growing body of scientists that strongly believes that we are being over-whelmed with free radicals and the only way to prevent free radical–based diseases, such as heart disease and cancer, is to take supplemental doses of antioxidant. They believe the antioxidants in our food are not in doses high enough to genuinely affect the progression of heart disease and cancer. Nevertheless, if you look at epidemiology work, there is no doubt that nations or communities consuming a significant amount of fruits and vegetables do have lower rates of heart disease and cancer, so even if it is not the antioxidants that is doing this, something is helping.

Well over half the adult population of any developed country has used some form of antioxidant-dose vitamin or herbal preparation in the pre-ceding month when any community is surveyed. This is despite the fact that no long-term clinical trial has ever been conducted to show a mor-tality benefit in healthy people taking antioxidant-dose vitamins. Mind you, there are over 6000 scientific papers appearing in medical literature to either directly or indirectly support the science behind antioxidants and quite a few convincing trials that show antioxidants do have a benefit. But this aside, there is still the possibility that the conservative medical world is right and vitamins don't work.

When I went through medical school there was no training in vitamin therapy, nor any specific nutritional training. I know this is changing and in the past five to 10 years the amount of nutritional training has increased. Still, the average doctor has no real knowledge of how vitamins, minerals and trace metals do their stuff; nor about the doses of vitamins or the combinations that are helpful in different types of diseases. The best way to hide a lack of knowledge on this when con-fronted with a patient asking questions is to say, 'Don't bother with all this stuff—it's complete rubbish.' Professional people who are alleged experts in an area do not like to admit that they have no knowledge so they tend to cover it up with comments such as this.

It may also be possible that doctors don't recommend vitamins because a script is not necessary. The script pad is what gives doctors 'power'. Anyone can walk into a health food store, chemist or supermarket, send off a form to a direct-mail company, or join any multi-level marketing company and get all manner of vitamins without anyone's permission. All you require is a name, an address and a credit card number. But if you want to start taking antibiotics or something to drop your blood pressure or lower your cholesterol, then you need permission from a doctor. Therefore, you have to make an appointment and pay the doctor money to obtain the pharmaceutical agent. Vitamins, however, are your own choice. A doctor derives no real benefit from your swallowing a vitamin, there is no real reason for him to know very much about it, nor be particularly interested.

Much of the education of the doctor these days is directly performed by drug reps or through pharmaceutical-sponsored education. Pharmaceutical companies on the whole do not make vitamins and have no real interest in vitamins being pushed forward as an alternative to their drugs. Pharmaceutical agents are certainly very effective agents. They are also very strong and usually very synthetic agents that have a marked metabolic effect on the body. Vitamins in antioxidant doses also have a metabolic effect on the body, but certainly without the same degree or strength of a pharmaceutical agent and, not surprisingly, without the same degree of side effects.

So armed with this caution regarding antioxidant vitamins, the next question is: what is the evidence for the benefits of antioxidants?

Antioxidant research

I started work as a doctor in 1979. In over 20 years of practice, I have seen many wonder drugs come and go on the market. I have attended many a lavish drug launch to be told of the wonderful properties of this drug and how it will revolutionise the treatment of that particular condition. When I returned to my practice and enthusiastically prescribed this drug I soon found out that not only did it not have the power I was expecting it to have, but it also had quite a few side effects. There is usually great enthusiasm in the first few months of using any drug but then most of us realise that what we'd been using in the past wasn't too bad after all, and any particular drug finds its own particular niche.

As I have just stated, drugs have strong metabolic effects and can have powerful side effects. Antioxidants, whether in food or in supplement form, are really nutritional therapy and not pharmacologic therapy. Unfortunately, most of the reasearch that has been done on antioxidant-dose vitamins by conservative researchers has been to use them as a drug and not as a nutritional supplement. When they don't get the same short-term large benefits that they see with a drug they then state the vitamin doesn't work.

When you are trialling any particular medical intervention, whether it is a drug, a surgical procedure, a vitamin, a herb or whatever, there are really five methods of assessment to decide whether this technique is going to be of any benefit:

1. laboratory evidence
2. animal experimentation
3. epidemiology studies
4. clinical trials
5. clinical experience.

LABORATORY EVIDENCE
There is no doubt that the common supplemental antioxidants—Vitamin E, Vitamin C and beta-carotene—perform their function. In the laboratory, these three substances have been clearly shown to be antioxidants—they are able to donate an electron to a free radical. This, however, does come at a price. If one of these antioxidants in isolation is overwhelmed by free radicals and donates all of its electrons, it becomes pro-oxidant and, therefore, a free radical. This is why it is so important not to just focus on one antioxidant.

Vitamin E, a fat-soluble vitamin that forms a protective shield around LDL cholesterol, temporarily becomes pro-oxidant (a free radical) once it donates one of its electrons. Vitamin C, a water-soluble molecule that hangs around in the bloodstream, is loaded with extra electrons and can donate the electron back to Vitamin E, returning Vitamin E to its original antioxidant state. The third line of defence is beta-carotene, which sits in the endothelial cell and the sub-interval space acting as an antioxidant, preventing the uptake of oxidised LDL cholesterol, thereby hopefully preventing the formation of a fatty plaque.

There is no doubt that the body has its own series of antioxidants as well, such as the chemical known as 'super-oxide dismutase' and another one known as 'glutathione', which work in conjunction with Vitamins E and C and beta-carotene to protect against free-radical attack.

ANIMAL EXPERIMENTATION

The great majority of studies performed on animals have been strongly supportive of the use of antioxidant-dose vitamins. If you feed a laboratory animal, such as a rat, a high processed diet for a few months, the rat rapidly develops atherosclerosis in the lining of its blood vessels within a few months. With an equivalent diet in human beings it might take somewhere between 20 and 40 years to induce the same disease.

A recent Vitamin E study in rats showed that the vitamin had a significant benefit in reducing the amount of atherosclerosis and fat build-up in the arteries by thinning the blood and reducing the free-radical attack through the Vitamin E as an antioxidant mechanism. The dual action of Vitamin E in being a blood thinner and also a strong antioxidant makes it an ideal antioxidant for use in vascular disease, such as heart attack and stroke.

In another study, looking at the major blood vessel coming off the heart in rabbits, it was found that oxidised LDL caused fatty plaques four times greater than unoxidised LDL. The addition of Vitamin E to the experiment resulted in an almost 50 per cent decrease in LDL in the plaques.

A group of monkeys on an atherosclerosis-inducing diet had less blockages in their arteries when given Vitamin E during a research study. In a group of monkeys that already had established blockages, there was a reduction of atherosclerosis from around 33 per cent to 8 per cent after eight months of treatment with Vitamin E.

EPIDEMIOLOGY STUDIES

Epidemiology is the study of populations. No attempt is made to control any variables within the population, unlike clinical trials. Data is collected throughout the study period and different variables are assessed.

One of the main facts derived from the Seven Countries Study was that the average intake of flavonoids were independent contributors in explaining the population differences in coronary heart disease mortality rates. Flavonoids are strong antioxidants present in tea, apples, onions and red wine. The more flavonoids you ingest, the less coronary heart disease and cancer you suffer. In this particular study, intake of vitamin supplements in the form of Vitamin E, beta-carotene and Vitamin C was not associated with any improvement in the coronary heart disease rates.

To date, around 25 epidemiology studies surveying well over 100 000 people have been performed. The majority of these studies showed a significant inverse relationship between the ingestion of Vitamin E, Vitamin C and beta-carotene, or the blood levels of these substances and the rates of heart disease and cancer.

One study in particular, which has now been progressing for the last 20 years, is the Nurses' Health Study from Boston. Around 87 000 nurses have been monitored for information regarding diet and supplement habits. In one branch of the study, the nurses taking a Vitamin E supplement somewhere between 100–500 units daily had a 41 per cent reduction in cardiac events.

Epidemiologic studies of Vitamin E levels and coronary heart disease

Study location	Sample/heart disease cases	Study findings	Date
Europe	12 populations	Inverse association between ischemic heart disease mortality and plasma Vitamin E levels	1989

India	595/72	Low plasma Vitamin E levels associated with an increased risk of coronary artery disease	1995
Finland	12 000/92	No consistent association between serum Vitamin E concentrations and risk of death from coronary artery disease	1985
Holland	10 532/106	No significant association between serum Vitamin E levels and risk of death from cardiovascular disease	1987
Turkey	133/62	Blood Vitamin E levels lower in patients with cardio-vascular disease	1995
Poland	131/53	Blood Vitamin E levels lower in angina patients	1991
Austria	200/100	Blood Vitamin E levels lower in angina patients	1997
United Kingdom	6000/110	Inverse association between plasma Vitamin E levels and risk of angina	1991
Sweden	99/64	Serum and LDL Vitamin E levels lower in patients with coronary artery disease	1996
United States	25 802/123	Decreased risk for subsequent MI with higher serum Vitamin E levels in subjects with high serum cholesterol levels	1994
Finland	5133/244	Decreased risk of heart disease in men and women in the highest tertile of Vitamin E intake	1994

A relatively recently reported study is the CPS-2 study (Cancer Prevention Study 2). In this particular study around 1 million Americans were monitored for seven years. It was shown that those people who supplemented with a combination of Vitamin E, Vitamin C and a multi-vitamin had an across-the-board 20 per cent reduction in all death, coronary heart disease and cancer. This benefit was not seen in the cigarette smokers in the study.

I would have to conclude that there is overwhelming epidemiologic evidence in support of the use of antioxidant vitamins and antioxidant foodstuffs in general as a means for preventing disease.

CLINICAL TRIALS

Here is where the trend seems to break down. The Holy Grail of the medical profession in terms of scientific information is the double-blind controlled clinical trial. This involves deciding on the parameter to be tested first. This parameter may be the use of a drug, vitamin or, at times, surgical procedure. The item is compared to a similar control group to see whether this procedure actually has any benefit. 'Blinding' the people in the trial does not mean poking their eyes out or destroying their retinas, but basically, if possible, stops them from knowing whether they are or are not having the active treatment.

One of my problems with these randomised trials is they often involve taking a population of, say, 30 000 to 40 000 people and weeding out the ones you don't want, ending up with about 5000 to 6000 people who suit what you're trying to achieve. This is certainly not representative of the general population and often quite large doses of pills are used to achieve the desired result. You can see clearly that this is a fairly artificial way of approaching a scientific principle, but it's basically the best way we've got.

Many doctors say all that vitamins do is give you expensive urine. US researchers—from Ann Arbor in Michigan, the University of California at San Diego and the University of Rochester in New York—demonstrated in a controlled clinical trial that a 12-week course of various combinations of Vitamin E, Vitamin C and beta-carotene showed a significant benefit in the antioxidant ability of the blood. Therefore, not only do vitamins give you 'expensive urine', they also give you 'expensive blood'—which is *exactly* what you want to happen. The doses that showed this significant improvement in antioxidant ability were 800 units of Vitamin E, 1000 milligrams of Vitamin C and 25 milligrams of beta-carotene.

I see the importance of this study in, firstly, highlighting the necessity for a particular dose. Many people will walk into a supermarket and pick up the cheapest vitamin (which is usually synthetic), swallow it for a few weeks and believe it will have benefit. Often, the vitamins are of sub-standard quality and the doses are too low. They certainly wouldn't have any benefits as antioxidants. Even worse than under-dosing with a probably useless, poor-quality vitamin, is the concept that 'more is better'. Taking mega-doses of vitamins without any medical supervision can also cause problems. I see no real justification in a healthy population, for example, going above a dose of 1000 units per day of Vitamin E. My suggested dose is somewhere between 400 and 800 units as a preventative. I have seen, in a minority of cases, a reversible multiple sclerosis–like syndrome in people taking more than 1500 units of Vitamin E each day.

Excessive doses of beta-carotene can cause the skin to go yellow as beta-carotene and its related compounds, the carotenoids, are substances that give colour to plants and protect plants against UV light. If we overdose with these substances from supplements or from taking in an excessive amount of carrots (carrots are high in beta-carotene and other carotenoids) we may suffer the consequences. Therefore, it is important that we all learn appropriate dosing schedules for vitamins.

This US study also highlighted the concepts of the antioxidant package. If you choose to supplement with antioxidants, it is important to take a 'package' rather than focusing on just one or two vitamins. Many of the trials of separate vitamins failed purely because they have only used one or two vitamins, usually in the wrong dose.

Vitamins are *not* drugs, but nutritional supplements. Because of the quality of our food these days, and the different nature of the diseases we are suffering, it is important to realise that vitamins should be taken on a regular, long-term basis. The study demonstrated that the benefits from vitamins are sustained over a three-month period. Other studies have shown that the effects of vitamins are also sustained over a much longer period.

THE EFFECT OF DIET ON ENDOTHELIAL FUNCTION

One of the world experts on the cardiovascular benefits of anti-oxidant vitamins is Professor Robert Vogel from the University of Baltimore in the US state of Maryland. He performed a study where researchers fed a group of healthy volunteers a breakfast from a popular takeaway food outlet and measured their endothelial function (the ability of the blood vessels to open under stress). As mentioned previously, this highly processed meal led to a 50 per cent reduction in endothelial ability. When half of the individuals were treated with 800 units of Vitamin E and 1000 milligrams of Vitamin C, the bad effect on endothelial function was completely prevented.

Professor Vogel went on to further experiment with different types of diet. Ten healthy volunteers with normal cholesterol levels were fed five different meals containing 50 grams of fat and a total of 900 kilocalories of energy.

The endothelial function was measured using a brachial artery technique before and three hours after each meal. The five meals were as follows:

1. 120 grams of non-preservative wholegrain bread with 50 grams of extra-virgin olive oil—basically high levels of mono-unsaturated fat and some processed carbohydrates.
2. 120 grams of non-preservative wholegrain bread with 50 grams of canola oil—a combination of moderate-level mono-unsaturated fat with plant-based Omega-3 polyunsaturated fat and the equivalent amount of processed carbohydrates.
3. 420 grams of canned red salmon with 30 grams of crackers—high-protein, high marine-based Omega-3 fatty acids and processed carbohydrates.

4. Identical to meal (1) with the addition of 1 gram of Vitamin C and 800 international units of Vitamin E—antioxidant-dose vitamins in supplement form.
5. Identical to meal (1) with the addition of 100 mls of balsamic vinegar and a salad of lettuce (1.5 cups), carrot (1 medium) and tomato (1 medium)—antioxidant-dose vitamins in food.

Only the first meal showed a reduction in endothelial function three hours after the meal. This reduction was just under one-third of normal, but still significant. All the other meals showed no deterioration in endothelial function, suggesting a strong benefit from antioxidants—whether in supplement or food form—and the Omega-3 fatty acids—whether derived from marine sources or from plants.

There have been numerous clinical trials looking at the rate of blockages in arteries using various doses of Vitamins E and C and beta-carotene. In one particular study, people who ingested above 100 units of Vitamin E daily demonstrated a reduced rate of progression of mild to moderate coronary blockages over a two-year period. In another recent trial of combination Vitamin E and Vitamin C, there was a *significant* (50 per cent) slowing of progression of disease in the carotid arteries (the blood flow to the brain).

With all this evidence, you are probably starting to ask, well, where is the big problem with vitamins? The big problem comes from looking at the long-term clinical results. The most important thing is what, in fact, happens to the people on a long-term basis when they swallow this stuff. Are they dying more quickly or developing some nasty disease without the vitamins? Or do vitamins show a significant benefit in terms of longevity, fewer heart attacks and less cancer? Unfortunately, in all of these areas the evidence is pretty thin on the ground either way.

In the early '90s, a study known as the ATBC Trial monitored some 29 000 Finnish males who had smoked 20 or so cigarettes a day for an average of 35 years. It followed these people for somewhere between five and eight years. They were given either 20 milligrams of synthetic beta-carotene, 50 milligrams of synthetic Vitamin E, both, or a placebo. There was no benefit in those receiving Vitamin E, but an 8 per cent higher mortality in the people receiving beta-carotene, plus a slight increase in lung cancer and cardiovascular disease.

A second study, known as the Caret Trial, showed no benefit from the combination of synthetic beta-carotene (30 milligrams per day) and 25 000 units of Vitamin A over placebos. The Caret Trial monitored 18 000 smokers, former smokers and asbestos workers over a four-year period. Of those who swallowed the supplements there was a 26 per cent higher rate of cardiovascular disease and lung cancer.

The response from the medical community to these trials has been ridiculous. These much-quoted trials are flawed and I believe they're a bit of a joke. Firstly, and most importantly, no-one could suggest that vitamins, which are useful adjuncts to a healthy lifestyle, could overcome the noxious effects of cigarette smoke. Secondly, the vitamins used in these trials were synthetic. At the least, synthetic vitamins are half as potent as natural vitamins, but at worst, because they are unnatural substances, they're very susceptible to becoming pro-oxidant (much more so than the natural versions). So when a person is overwhelmed by a noxious free radical–producing agent, such as a cigarette, and is given a weak synthetic vitamin at what I consider to be bizarre doses, it is no wonder the vitamins quickly become pro-oxidant and cause more harm than good.

To back up my argument, a group of 22 000 physicians in Boston, between 40 and 80 years of age were followed for an average of 12 years. They were given a very large dose of 50 milligrams beta-carotene on alternate days but had a very low incidence of smoking. There was no benefit or detriment in this group. Interestingly, 333 of the physicians with a history of stable heart disease revealed a 51 per cent reduction in further coronary events.

The only other negative trial of antioxidant vitamins in non-smokers on a blinded basis was a recent trial from Washington, DC, known as the HATS trial (HDL Atherosclerosis Treatment Study). It involved 160 men and women under the age of 70 with proven heart disease (either a prior heart attack, angina or stenting) and an abnormal angiogram. All of these people had low, good cholesterol levels. This trial went on for three years and had four groups. The first group were given Zocor (sim-vastatin, one of the statins) and niacin (a high dose of Vitamin B3 therapy). The dose of niacin was titrated to achieve a significant eleva-tion in HDL cholesterol without causing significant side effects, such as flushing. Group two were given antioxidant supplements. Group three were given a combination of cholesterol-lowering pills and antioxidants. Group four were given a placebo, or sugar pill. The antioxidants used in this situation were Vitamin C (500 milligrams twice daily), a natural Vitamin E (400 units twice daily), selenium (50 micrograms twice daily) and natural beta-carotene (12.5 milligrams twice daily).

The antioxidant vitamins appeared to block the HDL-raising effects of nicotinic acid. Also, looking at the results of the angiograms (dye study of the heart) that were performed after three years, the average blockages increased by around 4 per cent on no treatment, 2 per cent with antioxidants, 0.7 per cent with cholesterol-lowering treatment and antioxidants, and regressed by 0.4 per cent with the cholesterol-lowering treatment alone. One in four of the people on no treatment suffered some sort of cardiac event. (This is pretty standard for people with known siginficant heart disease over this period.) Twenty-one per cent on antioxidants alone suffered an event. This dropped back to 14 per cent in the group taking combined cholesterol-lowering therapy and antioxidants but only 3 per cent in the group taking the combined cho-lesterol-lowering therapy without antioxidants.

After these trials had been released, there was a furore in the medical profession with comments such as: 'Vitamin supplements dangerous in coronary heart disease', 'Complementary world proven wrong', and so on. There are a few points that need to be made here.

Firstly, the benefits of combined cholesterol-lowering therapy. Part of my reversal program is the use of a statin and niacin together. Standard therapy for atherosclerotic heart disease is usually just a statin, aspirin and maybe something else. Niacin is hardly ever used, despite the fact that there are now quite a number of trials that clearly show reversal of heart disease with a marked reduction in clinical events in those people who take these combined agents.

Although these trials do raise a concern around antioxidant-dose vitamins, I believe they should be taken in perspective. The Washington trial involved people with proven significant heart disease and low, good cholesterol levels. They represent somewhere between 20 and 30 per cent of the heart disease population. Therefore, these results cannot be extrapolated to other people with heart disease who do not have low HDL cholesterols, and certainly do not have much relevance to people who are not taking cholesterol-lowering pills. Should we damn all antioxidants because of this one particular trial? The answer is a definite '*no*'.

When you look further at this trial, it is more than likely that the high dose of beta-carotene blocked niacin's ability to raise HDL. This does not mean that Vitamin E and Vitamin C, or even selenium, should not be used with heart disease and niacin, but that we should avoid beta-carotene and niacin in combination.

Another concern I have is that I believe beta-carotene should not be used in doses above 15 milligrams a day. The trial that needs to be performed is a trial using varying doses of beta-carotene in conjunction with niacin to see whether the effects on HDL cholesterol are blocked. This seems absolute common sense to me. Unfortunately, most of the researchers involved with these trials, and the editorialists who wrote about the trials, seem to be missing this point.

These have been the only negative trials, but what about the neutral trials? To date there have been three trials that have shown no benefit or detriment from the use of antioxidant-dose vitamins. The first two have used Vitamin E alone and the last one, combinations of vitamins. The first trial to discuss has the rather bizarre name of the HOPE study, standing for Heart Outcomes Prevention Evaluation. It involved 9500 people aged 55 years or older with some sort of major risk factor for heart disease, established diabetes, or already having had some sort of vascular event. They monitored these people for around four-and-a-half years. Some were given Vitamin E, some were given a blood pressure drug known as ramipril, while some were given a sugar pill. At the end of the period, the blood pressure drug showed a 20 per cent reduction in heart attack death and stroke. The Vitamin E, which was 400 units of natural Vitamin E, did absolutely nothing. The headlines came out that Vitamin E was a 'fizzer'. Vitamin E had 'no benefit', etc.

The second trial was the Italian GISSI study, which involved just over 11 000 patients soon after they had had a heart attack. Some were given 1 gram of Omega-3 fish oil daily in capsule form, others were given 300 units of synthetic Vitamin E, still others were given both and some were given placebos. Their progress was monitored for three-and-a-half years. When the results were analysed, the treatment with the fish oil decreased the risk of death and heart attack and stroke, but overall, no significant benefit from the Vitamin E. When, however, the trial was re-examined looking at the individual components, Vitamin E had a 20 per cent lower risk for cardiovascular death and a 35 per cent lower risk for sudden death.

The final trial involved 20 000 patients in the United Kingdom, studied over a five-year period. They were treated with the cholesterol-lowering agent zocor, and given combinations of Vitamin E, Vitamin C and beta-carotene. This recently reported trial is known as the Heart Protection Study. In this trial there was no benefit or detriment from this therapy.

All of these trials are flawed in their design. As I have stated from the outset, vitamin therapy is an adjunct to a healthy lifestyle. Although lifestyle modification is given lip service by the people conducting the trials, there are no rigorous attempts to control which patients follow lifestyle advice and which patients do not. For example, in the HOPE trial the average weight of most of the people entering the trial was in the overweight range and did not change throughout the trial. In the GISSI trial there was a high proportion of smokers (commonly found in Europe) and the lifestyle modification was certainly not highlighted in the UK trial.

The HOPE trial evaluated single-vitamin therapy, but at least it was of a natural source and an appropriate dose. The trial only went for around four-and-a-half years which is far too short to see any significant benefit in this type of group, from Vitamin E. The GISSI trial used synthetic Vitamin E in a dose of 300 units per day, which is certainly not enough to expect any benefit, and I would not recommend the use of synthetic vitamins in the first place. Although the UK trial (the Heart Protection Study) used combinations of vitamins, I believe the dose of beta-carotene was far too high and the trial did not go for long enough, but the knock-out punch was that all the vitamins used were cheap synthetics!

What about the trials showing a positive benefit? There was a study performed in China on just under 30 000 rural citizens in the Linxian province. These people were probably nutritionally deficient. There were eight different combinations of vitamin supplements used with a significant reduction in cancer being shown, especially in the group taking beta-carotene, Vitamin E and selenium.

All the supporters of vitamin therapy have hung their hat on the study known as the CHAOS trial (standing for Cambridge Heart Antioxidant Study). It took a group of around 2000 people with proven heart disease (a secondary prevention trial) and treated half with between 400 and 800 units of natural Vitamin E. The average follow-up was just under two years and the treatment with Vitamin E showed a 40 per cent reduction in death and non-fatal heart attack. When looking at non-fatal heart attack alone there was a 77 per cent reduction. I must state that there is no drug that I'm aware of that is this powerful. The only other trial that came anywhere near this benefit was the Lyon Diet Heart Study, which showed a 75 per cent reduction in all death and all cardiac events on a diet. Strangely enough, there was no difference in overall death rate or fatal heart attack in CHAOS. One of the arguments for this was that there were not enough people in the trial to examine death over such a short period of time.

At this point I would like to explain what is known as 'intention to treat' in these trials. Once you commit yourself to one of these trials you are put into one of two groups: those using the vitamin or drug and those using the placebo. If, after a few months, you get sick of swallowing the pill and stop, your outcome is still considered as part of your initial group. Therefore, even if you weren't swallowing Vitamin E at the time, and died, the death was still attributable to Vitamin E. I know this sounds ridiculous, but unfortunately, this is how these trials work and why some of the information that comes from them is not accurate. In fact, when they looked further at all of the deaths in CHAOS, there were only six out of 72 deaths in people who were taking Vitamin E at the time. Therefore, 66 deaths out of 72 were in people not taking Vitamin E. This is statistically in favour of using Vitamin E.

Another rather dramatic study in a very high-risk group of people was a trial known as the SPACE Trial (Secondary Prevention with Anti-oxidants of Cardiovascular Disease in End Stage Renal Disease). They took a group of rather sick people with end-stage kidney failure and gave half of them high-dose Vitamin E (800 units of natural Vitamin E a day) and monitored them for just under two years. When they looked at the combination of heart attack, stroke or other vascular problems, there was a 54 per cent reduction, and a 70 per cent reduction in heart attack.

The results of the CHAOS and SPACE trials are difficult to compare with GISSI and HOPE. But, when you look at the annual rate of heart attack in the placebo (or sugar pill) groups in each of these trials, in HOPE and GISSI it was 3.8 and 2.5 per cent per year, whereas in CHAOS and SPACE, it was 5.1 and 12.3 per cent per year. The point I am making is that the CHAOS and SPACE groups were a much higher-risk group and therefore stood to benefit with these shorter-term trials.

Another interesting point is the particular group in the studies. For example, CHAOS was performed in the United Kingdom, where they have never really been known to be world champions in dietary discretion. The antioxidant content of the British diet is not particularly high, therefore, in people at high risk you would expect benefit from the addition of a natural antioxidant. Moving to the GISSI trial, the antioxidant content of the Italian diet is much higher, therefore, the people who did not respond particularly well to Vitamin E alone may have been reisistant to antioxidant treatment in the first place as they had already had a heart attack despite being on a Mediterranean-style diet.

I am a strong believer that we should all be supplementing with a sensible antioxidant regimen. I do, however, admit that there has never been an adequate trial of antioxidant-dose vitamins performed in healthy people. For a trial to adequately show that antioxidant vitamins are of benefit over and above a healthy lifestyle you need at least 30 000 to 50 000 people monitored for somewhere between 15 and 20 years. The closest we have come to this have been observational trials such as CPS-2 and the Nurses' Health Study.

The argument that people inclined to take vitamins are more likely to live a healthy lifestyle assumes that vitamins are more a marker of a healthy lifestyle than a cause of any benefit by themselves. My argument against this is that if you look at most dietary interventions combined with other lifestyle modifications, there is usually only somewhere between a 10 and 15 per cent benefit in terms of mortality and death rate; whereas, CPS-2 showed a 20 per cent reduction across the board in those taking vitamins, and the Nurses' Health Study showed a 40 per cent reduction in those taking Vitamin E for cardiac events.

I am also not so foolish to suggest that vitamins are a panacea. There are many people who are still sprightly and enjoying their lives in their nineties but have never been anywhere near a health food store or a vitamin. There are also quite a few people who have swallowed vitamins religiously for many years and have succumbed to major diseases. There will always be exceptions to the rule, but, personally, I have seen dramatic results from the use of sensible vitamin therapy when combined with proper lifestyle principles.

The second area to consider when discussing vitamins is the type of vitamins used. Firstly, and most importantly, not all vitamins are the same. It is very difficult for members of the public to know whether they are taking good-quality vitamins or not. The following are some important hints along these lines:

- When considering Vitamin E, the natural form is d-alpha-tocopherol. If the side of the bottle says 'dl-alpha-tocopherol' you know you are taking synthetic alpha-tocopherol and I would advise against using this supplement.
- In the case of beta-carotene, if it does not specifically say 'natural beta-carotene', but just 'beta-carotene' alone, it is likely that the beta-carotene comes from a synthetic source. I would have trepidations swallowing synthetic beta-carotene, especially at high

doses. If the label says 'beta-carotene (D.Salina)', it is the natural form of beta-carotene derived from algae. (The major harvesting areas for D. Salina algae in the world are, in fact, in Australia.) This natural form of beta-carotene contains five of the six major natural carotenoids that are important for human health. I will discuss these later.

Some of the doses in these clinical trials have been ridiculous. They are either too high or too low. They also use the wrong combinations of drugs. Single vitamin therapy is of no real benefit—it often renders that vitamin pro-oxidant when it is attacked by a free radical and therefore makes the vitamin therapy less than useful. Some of the more creative companies are now providing excellent coverage with the broad spectrum of vitamins, requiring the ingestion of only one to three pills twice daily.

The next specific problem is that there will be some interaction between drugs and vitamins. About a year ago a study came out stating that Gingko and Aspirin together could cause serious bleeding. Well, guess what—this is part of both of their actions, so together the blood does become even thinner. Obviously, if someone is taking these drugs and herbs separately or in combination, their blood will be thinner than that of someone who is not taking them. If this person then happens to go in for an emergency surgical procedure, there is no doubt they have a greater chance of bleeding during and after the procedure. Does this then give the researchers the right to suggest Gingko is dangerous?

I have no doubt that in the Washington trial, where vitamins blunted the benefits of the cholesterol-lowing therapy, this was a specific inter-action between high-dose beta-carotene and nicotinic acid. This does not mean we should throw out the baby with the bath water and suggest all vitamins may be dangerous for patients with heart disease. All it means is we should do further research to look at the interaction between certain vitamins and particular cholesterol-lowering therapy. This would not be a difficult trial to perform and should be done as soon as possible.

Another major criticism of most of these trials is the length of study. Pharmaceutical drugs are much stronger agents with, of course, more side effects. Because pharmaceutical drugs are so strong, they need fewer people studied for a shorter period of time. Vitamins do not have the same power as pharmaceutical drugs (nor the same side effects) and are a useful adjunct to a healthy lifestyle. Therefore, to prove a definite benefit from taking vitamins we need more people studied for a longer time.

The blinded or controlled trials showing a proven efficacy were in those people at very high risk. In other trials, such as CHAOS, HOPE and GISSI, the people were either at lower risk (as seen by the lower heart attack and death rates in the control groups), the wrong group to study in the first place, or on synthetic vitamins. Also, in these groups there were no strong efforts to modify lifestyle factors.

This brings me to my final point, which is the ridiculous nature of some of these trials in studying the wrong type of people. One of the arguments against the GISSI trial in Italy is that the people eat a diet already high in antioxidants so they are probably resistant to any anti-oxidant therapy. These people have been given the unfortunate term of the RANCIDS. Maybe the different genetics and the different environmental factors such as the amount of antioxidants in the diet, the amount of pollution in the air, other background nutritional and lifestyle factors may affect the outcomes of particular trials.

Most ridiculous, however, is to study adjunctive nutritional therapy, such as antioxidant vitamins, in people with poor lifestyle behaviours. There is no point giving vitamins to cigarette smokers (such as the ATBC and Caret trials) or to expect that vitamins will have much benefit to people who continue to be overweight (such as the HOPE trial). For all these reasons, I think it is obvious that I have been disappointed to date, not so much with the results of the trial, but with the manner in which these trials have been designed and conducted. Even worse than this are the somewhat spurious conclusions that have been made from these trials without thinking laterally about the possibilities of why the trials are not working.

CLINICAL EXPERIENCE
Despite all this carry-on about evidence-based medicine and scientific proof, the ongoing subjectivity of our world never fails to astound me.

I was in Orlando, Florida, in 2001 for the American College of Cardiology meeting. At that meeting I heard one of the world experts on antioxidants, Professor David Harrison, give an excellent summary of the science behind free radical and antioxidant interaction. At the end of the lecture he had a throwaway slide implying Vitamin E was of no real benefit and could possibly even cause harm. Professor Harrison said recently that evidence is now showing that vitamins should not be used alone, and the combination of Vitamin E and Vitamin C has been shown to cause a 50 per cent reduction in the progression of vascular disease in one particular study. This shows great promise for future vitamin research. Why the turnaround?

In my practice I have seen far too many patients who appear to look 10 to 15 years younger than their stated age. They then tell me they have been on antioxidant-dose vitamins for many years. I have seen people who should have vicious heart disease on their risk factor profile but, again, when I check them with high-speed CT scanning of the heart, they have minimal or no evidence of any vascular disease whatsoever. These people attribute their well-being to good lifestyle principles and antioxidant-dose vitamins.

Eighty per cent of the medicine we practise every day is experience-based medicine, not evidence-based medicine. Although there is a strong place in our modern world with our modern technology for evidence-based medicine, we should not lose sight of the importance of experience. The 'sixth sense' in medicine is becoming progressively lost in technology and, interestingly, with this increase in technology comes an increasing suspicion of the medical profession. The decision to take a cholesterol-lowering pill is really not yours; it does come down to whether you are prepared to swallow the pill that has been prescribed, but you must get permission from a doctor to take this pill in the first place. The decision, however, to use antioxidant-dose vitamins is entirely yours, whether your doctor does or doesn't condone it.

My attitude to this is very straightforward. The information regarding vitamin therapy, although confusing, is certainly *out there* and I believe it is up to you as the intelligent consumer to read the information and decide which way you would like to go. In my mind, there is no doubt from the totality of evidence that a poor lifestyle will lead to a poor outcome in most cases. There is also no doubt from the totality of evidence that following Cell Factor therapy without the ingestion of antioxident-dose vitamins will give you a much better chance of a long and healthy life. If you want the optimum benefit from Cell Factor therapy, I believe it is important to follow the principles detailed in this book, which include the sensible ingestion of antioxidant-dose vitamins.

Types of antioxidants

I have already mentioned how antioxidants neutralise free radicals. The only question in science is not whether this is the case (as we all agree that it does) but what types of antioxidants are most beneficial in performing these functions. In a natural environment where all of our exposures every day are natural exposures, we would only need natural solutions. But today we certainly need extra doses of natural antioxidants—which, unfortunately, we cannot provide from our diets—to combat the excessive load of free radicals.

There are five sources of antioxidants:

1. fruit and vegetables
2. tea
3. extra-virgin olive oil
4. red wine
5. antioxidant-dose vitamins.

You don't need a Nobel prize to know fruits and vegetables are good for you. There are some proponents of the high-protein, low-carbohydrate diet who actually state that fruit and vegetables (especially excessive amounts of fruit) contribute to insulin resistance and diabetes. There is not one shred of scientific evidence for this rather bizarre comment.

Fruit and vegetables contain over 600 naturally occurring antioxidants. The carbohydrate in fruit and vegetables is often in the form of fibre—which has also been shown to significantly benefit diabetes sufferers and people with vascular disease, and also some studies suggest a reduction in cancer. The Seven Countries Study showed that nations where high levels of fruit and vegetables are consumed, such as Greece and Italy, have lower rates of vascular disease than nations where there was a low consumption, such as Finland. In fact, the rates of heart attack in Crete were 30 times lower than in Finland. I'm not suggesting that this is all due to the fruit and vegetable intake.

There are five main groups of nutrients in plants, known as phyto-nutrients. These are:

1. phyto-sterols
2. glutathione and other sulphur compounds
3. flavonoids/terpenoids
4. carotenoids
5. other vitamins and minerals.

PHYTO-STEROLS

Humans are a funny lot. We believe the best form of medical therapy comes from a pill or a surgical procedure. If a scientist finds a particular compound in nature and it's put into a food product you can buy off the shelf, more value is placed on the medical claim written on the side of the packet than on the pot-pourri of whole fruits and vegetables that are available. Nothing proves this more than the new 'wonder margarines', which lower cholesterol.

In the late '90s these new margarines exploded on to the market. Anyone who had been inducted into the cholesterol hall of fame was rushing out to their local supermarket to purchase a tub. The scenes were reminiscent of the New Year sales. I am in no way demeaning the benefits of these margarines—there is somewhere between a 10 and 15 per cent reduction in LDL (bad) cholesterol if they are used regularly. The important point to note, however, is that these substances are abundant in fruits and vegetables.

The substances are known as phyto-sterols. The most abundant sterol is, of course, cholesterol, a vital substance for many reactions within the body and, in particular, for the building of our cell membranes and

many of our steroid hormones. However, as we know, excessive cholesterol can spill into fatty plaques and contribute to atherosclerosis.
Nature knew this long before the multinational food companies did
and, in fact, included phyto-sterols in our diet naturally to ensure we
did not take in excessive amounts of cholesterol. These plant sterols
compete for cholesterol absorption in the gut. You can derive exactly the
same benefit from eating half an avocado a day as you will from using
cholesterol-lowering margarine. If you study the plant kingdom you'll
find many plants (not just avocados) containing significant amounts of
plant sterols, such as soy beans, legumes and cucumbers.

GLUTATHIONE AND OTHER SULPHUR COMPOUNDS

Glutathione is one of the important internal antioxidant systems.
Sulphur is an important component of glutathione and, in fact, is found
in many of the protective chemical reactions within the body. We need
glutathione to ensure our metabolic system works as it is supposed to.

Rich sources of glutathione are cabbage, garlic, onions, broccoli, cau-
liflower and, I hate to admit this . . . brussels sprouts. Although I have
no doubt as to the benefits of brussels sprouts, I'm afraid I was trauma-
tised as a child by being forced to eat one and I think brussels sprouts
prove that God does have a sense of humour.

FLAVONOIDS/TERPENOIDS

The sources of flavonoids are citrus fruit, onions, apples, grapes, wine,
tea and chocolate. Unfortunately, when I make comments like this,
people will focus on something like chocolate, rush off and start consuming it by the tonne, believing, because it is high in flavonoids, it has
enormous benefits. You must also remember that chocolate is high in
processed carbohydrate and also has a bit of saturated fat and trans fatty
acids thrown in for good measure. Remember, the whole package of the
food is what needs to be considered.

There are five major groups of flavonoids:

- proanthacyanidins
- polyphenols

- isoflavones
- quercetins
- citrus bioflavonoids.

Proanthacyanidins: Proanthacyanidins are especially found in grape-seed or pine-bark extracts. One of the pieces of advice I give to anyone regarding nutrition is: 'If you can eat the seed, eat it!' Rather than spitting out a grape seed, my advice is to chew on the seed and break it up, as you will be releasing the extracts of the seed directly and derive enormous benefits. Grape-seed and pine-bark extracts are now available in supplement form.

There are no long-term clinical trials as to the benefits of these extracts but there are numerous anecdotal reports of improvements in all manner of illnesses in people taking some form of proanthacyanidins. I have had numerous people come up to me after my lectures telling me how their life was turned around when they started taking some form of grape-seed or pine-bark extract. Of course, I'm not suggesting, as a medical scientist, that this is definite proof of their action, but I must say I have seen some dramatic results. In laboratory work, these substances have been shown to be anywhere between 20 and 50 times more potent that Vitamin C and Vitamin E. I would put the proanthacyanidins in the 'super antioxidant' category. I certainly take these substances myself. I admit, though, they are expensive and the scientific work behind them is not as strong as it is for Vitamins C and E and carotenoid compounds.

> **Case study**—I well recall the case of a young girl who had attended one of my lectures. Three months after the lecture she told me she had an addiction to painkillers because of a dreadful condition known as fibro myalgia, which causes intense pain in the muscles. After she heard me talking about the benefits of proanthacyanidins, she began taking one of these substances. Within three months she was off all painkillers and able to attend school for the first time in 12 months.

Polyphenols: There have been numerous studies supporting the use of substances high in polyphenols as a method of reducing the risk for common diseases. Polyphenols are very strong antioxidants and are found in red wine, extra-virgin olive oil and tea.

In the '70s, a study showed a strong protective benefit from the use of black tea. A recent study from the Netherlands showed the risk of dying from heart disease was significantly lower in those who had a high consumption of tea. Another study from Norway showed a 36 per cent reduction in coronary disease in tea-drinkers compared with those who did not drink tea. A Welsh study, however, suggested a higher intake of white tea was associated with an increased risk of heart disease. In this particular study, the participants tended to be smokers who drank less alcohol and consumed more bad fat. One of the more ridiculous explanations for the study's results was that milk protein prevented the absorption of different components of tea. Other studies have clearly shown that milk has no effect on the absorption of the flavonoids, quercetin and catechin. In studies in Japan, the population in areas where green tea is produced has much lower rates of heart disease and cancer than the rest of Japan.

The mechanisms actions of the antioxidants in tea can be summarised as follows:

- Tea has no appreciable effect on cholesterol levels.
- The antioxidants in tea work at the blood-vessel wall, not on LDL, as the polyphenols are water-soluble and not fat-soluble.
- The antioxidants in tea have been shown to have a significant anti-inflammatory component, which has increasingly been shown to be important in heart disease.

There is a strong association between chronic infections, such as Chlamydia Pneumoniae, a virus known as CMV (cytomegalo virus), and even the bug that causes peptic ulcers, Helicobacter, and an increase in the degree of antherosclerosis. It is felt that these bacteria may cause the fat build-up in the lining of the arteries to accelerate through inflammatory mechanisms. Therefore, enjoying a simple cup of tea a few times a day may contribute to suppressing this inflammatory response. This is one of the proposed mechanisms whereby tea, and especially its polyphenolic components, can fight inflammation.

Finally, one of the major components of heart disease is thrombosis (a tendency towards clotting). Clotting occurs because of a combination of clotting factors, which are proteins combining with platelets, the sticky cells in the bloodstream. Once these platelets are activated they combine with the clotting proteins to form a clot. If there is an excessive switching on of this sytsem, excessive clotting occurs. Again, the simple enjoyment of a cup of tea can release these polyphenols into the bloodstream, preventing platelets from being activated, thus keeping the blood 'thin'. Therefore tea has wonderful substances that assist in the prevention of heart disease and cancer through many mechanisms.

Regardless of the science, the next time you enjoy a cup of tea, not only savour the flavour—so to speak—but quietly realise what other enormous benefits each sip is affording you. The study from the Netherlands followed 806 men between the ages of 65 and 84. It found those who had the highest intake of catechins (a flavonoid found in tea, apples and chocolate) had 51 per cent less heart disease over a 10-year period. That old adage of 'An apple a day keeps the doctor away' may be absolutely true! These magic catechins are about 30 per cent of the dry weight of green tea and about 9 per cent of black tea. Obviously, green tea is better for you than black tea but, between you and me, I find the stuff rather unpalatable. If you are one of those lucky people who enjoys green tea, keep drinking it because it's good for you.

'Hang on a minute,' you say, 'you also mentioned *chocolate*!' Am I going to give all you chocoholics carte blanche to run out there and swallow any piece of chocolate you desire because you know it is good for you? The answer to this is 'Of course not!' Although I don't think it hurts to have a little bit of chocolate every now and then, as I mentioned before there is such a high proportion of trans fatty acids and carboyhydrates in chocolate. It is better to keep consumption of this down to a minimum—but like everything in life, balance is probably the best approach.

What about coffee? Over the past 30 to 40 years we have had almost every foodstuff, beverage or supplement implicated in most diseases. There have been over 500 reports on the health benefits or detriments of coffee and I must state that, up to now, most of the evidence is quite conflicting. But forget about the health benefits or detriments for a second . . . those of us who enjoy our coffee should be happy to admit it is something we look forward to every day. I only started drinking coffee a few years ago, but am more than happy to admit I look forward to one or two cups of good-quality espresso coffee each day. Frankly, I am not particularly perturbed by some 'possible link' between such a daily dose of coffee and health. In fact, the more I research the area, the more I realise coffee in moderation is similar to alcohol in moderation. In low doses it is probably good for you.

There is no doubt that coffee has the highest content of caffeine of all food and beverages. It is a proven stimulant, and I, like many others, know that if I have coffee after a certain hour in the evening, I find it difficult to sleep. Equally, many other people can drink coffee and it has absolutely no effect on their sleeping patterns. Let's look at some of the coffee studies published.

Firstly, caffeine in moderation has been shown to reduce asthma. I would certainly not suggest coffee should be a replacement for effective anti-asthma treatment, but in asthma sufferers there is no doubt that enjoying a few cups of coffee a day may assist in their long-term management.

Coffee drinking during the day while you are driving (not literally, of course) can also help increase alertness and mood, and may combat driver sleepiness. Some studies have suggested a relationship between coffee consumption and reduced levels of depression and anxiety.

A recent study, known as the Male Health Professional Study, monitored 45 000 males over a 10-year period. It showed that men who consumed a few cups of coffee a day had less renal stones and a graded decrease in gallstones over the same period of time. One cup a day reduced the risk of gallstones by 20 per cent; two to three cups a day of caffeinated coffee led to a 40 per cent lower risk of gallstone development; and four or more cups a day, a 45 per cent lower risk of gallstones. No benefit was shown with decaffeinated coffee.

There is a rather weak association between coffee consumption and reduced risk for colon cancer, but certainly no studies suggest an increase in risk. The most interesting evidence comes from the association between coffee consumption and heart disease. In people drinking instant coffee, there are two substances, cafestol and kahwheol, that tend to raise cholesterol levels. Consuming more than four cups of instant coffee a day can increase the cholesteol level anywhere between 0.5 to 1.2 millimoles per litre. The use of filtered or espresso coffee, however, filters out these cholesterol-raising substances. In fact, in long-term studies, such as the Male Health Professional Study, the Nurses' Health Study or the Scottish Health Study, there is no increase in cardiovascular risk and coffee consumption. In another study, known as the John Hopkins Precursor Study, consuming more than five cups of coffee a day showed a three times increased risk for heart disease.

One of the interesting findings is that there appears to be more risk for raising cholesterol from drinking decaffeinated coffee, as opposed to normal, so there is probably no benefit in switching to 'decaf'. Two recent studies have shown that consuming more than four cups of coffee a day may increase the homocysteine levels, which are also associated with heart disease.

In my opinion, the evidence for consuming daily more than four cups of any type of coffee may be associated with some elevation in cholesterol levels and some possible cardiovascular harm, but there are certainly no problems whatsoever with the moderate consumption of coffee—especially good-quality filtered or espresso coffee. I know that I will continue to enjoy this as part of my normal day.

Isoflavones: The isoflavones in soy products are known as genistein and dadizein. These products are known as phyto-oestrogens. Some authorities consider phyto-oestrogens to be selective oestrogen receptor modulators (SORMS or SERMS—depending on which country you come from and which way you spell oestrogen). The interesting and important aspect of SORMS is that in some situations they can act as weak oestrogen stimulators, and in other situations they may block the effect of oestrogen.

In women with high oestrogen levels, the ingestion of soy proteins (and therefore, isoflavones) may reduce the more concerning effects of high levels of oestrogen, such as predisposition for breast cancer. In other situations, such as the post-menopausal female who loses her oestrogen secretion, the isoflavones can have a weak stimulatory effect and, therefore, have the potential to reduce many of the peri- and post-menopausal problems, such as the symptoms of menopause—flushing, irritability, mood swings, osteoporosis and cardiovascular disease.

Isoflavones also have antioxidant properties, inhibiting LDL cholesterol and other aspects of the generation of atherosclerosis, such as endothelial dysfunction and smooth muscle cell proliferation. A relatively recent study also showed an added benefit of isoflavone therapy. Isoflavones derived from red clover in a dose of 40 milligrams a day demonstrated a 28 per cent increase in HDL cholesterol. Isoflavones have also been shown to reduce osteoporosis, and genistein, in particular, has suggested anti-tumour activity in some promising work.

The data suggest that a sensible consumption of soy products in the form of tofu and milk, and even its addition to energy bars, breakfast cereals, breads and pasta, may be of significant benefit to the general population. The isoflavones are present in soy protein in a dose of 1 to 3 milligrams for each gram of protein. The typical suggested serving is somewhere between 25 and 40 milligrams of isoflavones. Many of the commercial preparation tablets of isoflavone contain 40 milligrams.

Quercetins: Quercetins are a group of antioxidants present in red wine and tea, but are also available in supplement form. I will discuss alcohol separately.

Citrus bioflavonoids: Citrus fruits across the board have many wonderful phyto-chemicals that promote good health. We all associate the ingestion of oranges with Vitamin C, but oranges and other citrus fruits are wonderful sources of citrus bioflavonoids, which are part of the general exogenous (external) antioxidant system that promotes good health in our body. The next time you feel like something to eat, reach for an orange or one of the other citrus fruits. I can promise you it's a lot better for you than a biscuit or some so-called 'energy bar'.

CAROTENOIDS

There are around 600 different types of carotenoids found in fruits and vegetables. Carotenoids are largely responsible for giving specific plants their colourings, but they have many other amazing properties that promote good health.

There are six major carotenoids found in our bloodstream and tissues in appreciable quantities. These include beta-carotene, alpha-carotene, lutein, zeaxanthin, cryptoaxanthin and lycopene. It is important to note that the absorption of carotenoids in most cases is improved after cooking. The presence of protein, dietary fat and Vitamin E all increase the absorption of carotenoids.

Carotenoids are found in the following foods:

- Alpha- and beta-carotene
  - Carrots
  - Pumpkins
  - Apricots
  - Rockmelon
  - Leafy green vegetables
  - Sweet potato
  - Winter squash
- Lutein
  - Leafy green vegetables
  - Pumpkins
  - Red peppers
- Zeanthin
  - Mangoes
  - Nectarines
  - Oranges, mandarins, tangerines
  - Pawpaw
  - Peaches

- Cryptoanthin
  - Mangoes
  - Nectarines
  - Oranges, mandarins, tangerines
  - Pawpaw
  - Peaches
- Lycopene
  - Cooked tomato
  - Tomato sauce
  - Tomato paste
  - Guava
  - Pink grapefruit
  - Watermelon.

You will note that it is the yellow and dark green vegetables that contain the higher concentration of carotenoids.

There is a distinction between synthetic and naturally occurring carotenoids. Synthetic carotenoids contain only beta-carotene in the trans-configuration. Natural beta-carotene has a mixture of all of the carotenoids mentioned and recent research has shown natural beta-carotene substances are a much more efficient antioxidant than synthetic beta-carotene.

A great majority of the commercial, natural beta-carotene source is produced in Australia. There are two large algae farms cultivating the D.Salina algae, which is a rich source of natural carotenoids. Of course, it is preferable to obtain all of your carotenoids from yellow and dark green vegetables, but it certainly does not hurt to obtain a small dose of supplemental carotenoids somewhere in the 6–12-milligram range from supplements. As I have stressed throughout the book, read the labels and ensure the source of beta-carotene is natural. The best way to do this is to see if it reads (after the fine print), 'Beta-carotene natural source—D.Salina'.

There has been some scaremongering regarding beta-carotene in the medical literature because of two studies performed on cigarette smokers. It was found that long-term cigarette smokers who took synthetic beta-carotene had a slightly higher risk of lung cancer. This is no surprise to me as, firstly, synthetic beta-carotene is an extremely weak antioxidant and when a very powerful oxidant, such as cigarette smoke, is introduced into the body, this quickly changes the weak antioxidant to another pro-oxidant substance, which works in concert with cigarette smoke to cause problems. The simple answer here is, don't smoke. In another study of non-smokers, known as the Male Physicians' Trial, there was no harm from taking synthetic beta-carotene. There was also no benefit—which, again, is of no surprise as I do not believe synthetic vitamins should be taken.

The third piece of scaremongering came from a group in Washington, DC, that used combination vitamins in addition to a statin cholesterol-lowering agent and nicotinic acid (or niacin). It showed the multi-vitamin combination blunted the beneficial effects of the cholesterol-lowering agents. This was using natural beta-carotene and in a dose of 25 milligrams per day, which I believe is too high a dose. There was a specific interaction between beta-carotene and nicotinic acid which blunted the effect of nicotinic acid. The conclusion came out that antioxidant vitamins may do harm but in reality, this was a specific drug–vitamin interaction. For this reason, I believe the study was of no real value apart from its ability to highlight this particular problem.

How then, do carotenoids work? Like all vitamins, carotenoids are a 'package' that work together with a diverse number of biologic actions.

Vitamin A is a fat-soluble vitamin that is essential for many reactions, especially in the immune system and the skin. One of the problems, however, is that Vitamin A by itself can be quite toxic and it is never quite clear what is a safe dose. A recent study in the elderly suggested that excess Vitamin A from supplements may contribute to osteoporosis. If you supplement, I would avoid doses higher than 5000 international units of Vitamin A. There have been some concerns regarding the use of Vitamin A, for example, in pregnancy and its effects on the foetus. Beta-carotene, however, in its natural form, will be converted to Vitamin A only when the body needs a particular amount of that vitamin. Alpha-carotene and cryptoxanthin also have some pro–Vitamin A characteristics.

The carotenoids as a group are very effective antioxidants. Lycopene is the strongest of all the carotenoids. It is found in very high proportions in tomato-based products—especially cooked tomatoes, tomato paste and tomato sauce. Lycopene has very specific anti-cancer actions, especially in regard to prostate cancer, and to some degree, breast cancer. The carotenoids also prevent free-radical damage from not only cancer, but also premature ageing, atherosclerosis and age-related eye diseases. Carotenoids are very effective immune stimulants. They have been shown to inhibit the proliferation of growth of cancer cells.

Carotenoids colour plants to protect them from UV radiation. They can also protect humans from UV radiation, reducing the risk for skin cancer and sun-induced skin damage. Lutein and zeaxanthin are specific carotenoids for vision. There is now a significant body of scientific work supporting the use of antioxidants and, in particular, these two carotenoids, in preventing or reducing age-related eye disease such as macular degeneration and cataracts.

Lycopene and beta-carotene are important substances in regulating the local communication from cell to cell. Without this local communication, it is impossible for the cellular neighbourhood to coordinate its normal production response to wear and tear and external trauma.

There is no real recommended daily allowance for carotenoid intake. The recommended dietary intake for Vitamin A is 1000 retinol equivalents (RE) for men and 800 in women. One RE equals 1 microgram of retinol, which equals 6 micrograms of beta-carotene, which in turn equals 12 micrograms of other pro–Vitamin A carotenoids. A typical Western diet contains somewhere between 1.5 and 3 milligrams of beta-carotene, and 3.5 and 7.5 milligrams of total carotenoids. You cannot assume, just because you have a few fruits and vegetables every day, that you will be getting significant amounts of carotenoids. For example, a diet containing broccoli, carrots, tomatoes and watermelon will give you significant doses of beta-carotene and the other carotenoids, but a diet of apples, pears, potatoes and corn will give minimal amounts of carotenoids and certainly nowhere near the recommended intake. As with all recommended daily intakes, the amount suggested is enough to prevent a deficiency disease. There has been no suggested dose to function as an antioxidant to prevent our common killers: heart disease and cancer.

So what evidence has been published suggesting that carotenoids are of any value? There are now over 40 epidemiologic studies totalling 20 000 patients with up to 20 years' follow-up that show that the highest intake of carotenoids in the diet, or in the bloodstream, is associated with the lowest cancer risk. Across the studies there has been up to a 60 per cent reduction in cancer risk with the highest carotenoid intake or blood levels. The controlled clinical trials have not been as forthcoming.

A five-year trial from China, known as the Linxian Trial, showed that a combination of supplemental synthetic beta-carotene, Vitamin C and selenium in a group of 30 000 individuals, who were probably nutritionally deficient to start with, led to a 9 per cent decrease in death and a 13 per cent decrease in cancer. The other trials I have mentioned that assessed the effects of synthetic beta-carotene in very high doses in smokers showed a slightly higher rate of lung cancer.

The associations of carotenoids and coronary heart disease, however, are even more striking. The highest intakes and blood levels of carotenoids showed a decrease in the risk for coronary heart disease. There have been around 100 000 people studied showing between 29 and 50 per cent reduced rate of heart disease. I must state, however, that there have been no long-term studies using natural carotenoid supplements to show a benefit or detriment of these agents in the prevention of heart disease or cancer. All of the studies that have been performed have shown a benefit with the use of natural foods containing the carotenoids. It may be some, as yet, unknown substance also in these foods that are high in carotenoids which has the protective effects. It may be much smaller doses of this unknown substance causing the enormous reduction in heart disease and cancer.

I am not convinced there will ever be any decent study performed on a long-term basis for any type of supplement. The reality is there are no randomised clinical trials of dietary therapy over the long term. Nobody really knows whether 15 to 30 years of eating in a particular way does or does not have a long-term benefit. All of the assumptions made from dieting come from epidemiological studies where there are many other confounding factors. For example, the people on Crete and Okinawa (whose lifestyle and diet has been mentioned on a few occasions throughout this book) have something very much in common: the fact that these are more isolated communities and on islands. It may be the smaller population and the lesser amounts of pollution, along with more reliance on the legs as a form of transport rather than automobiles, that have the most profound effect on longevity.

All we can really say at this stage is that all of the indirect evidence points towards one particular eating habit or one particular group of foodstuffs, such as carotenoids, as being beneficial. As our foods increasingly become more synthetic, we are missing out on many of these natural food components, and the next best alternative is to supplement with the natural concentrates.

The final question we should ask is: are carotenoids safe? Apart from the caveats regarding the use of synthetic beta-carotene and smokers, the long-term safety data of carotenoids appear very sound. The most common problem seen with the intake of high levels of carotenoids (greater than 30 milligrams a day) is a syndrome known as carotenaemia, which is a yellow discolouration of the skin. This is completely reversible when the high levels of carotenoids are reduced. Carotenaemia is commonly seen in people eating excessive amounts of carrots—in particular, people drinking carrot juice at high doses on a regular basis.

As I have suggested before, it is my belief that carotenoid supplements should be taken in their natural form, most commonly from the D.Salina algae source in a dose somewhere between 6 and 12 milligrams of carotenoid a day.

OTHER VITAMINS AND MINERALS
Vitamins, minerals and trace metals are best obtained from natural sources, i.e. food. There is a concept known as 'bio-availability'. This is

the amount of any substance taken in food, supplement or pill that actually ends up inside the body after digestion. The most bio-available vitamins working at the tissue level are those that are incorporated into foodstuffs and not made in a synthetic laboratory somewhere.

There are a number of very clever vitamin companies now concentrating vitamins in food either using baker's yeast or even growing the vitamins incorporated into fruits and vegetables. Many of these companies have developed excellent techniques so that not only are you taking an antioxidant dose of vitamin, but you are also ingesting the added benefit of the phyto-chemicals from the food source used. These supplements tend to be expensive and, again, there are no clinical trials to say whether these vitamins have a significant benefit over the synthetic vitamins. I believe a decision has to be made as to whether you take vitamins at all and, if you are going to spend your money, I would suggest you spend your money on the better quality of vitamins rather than the cheaper synthetics, which I believe have a potential for harm rather than for the good derived from using the natural source vitamins—especially those incorporated with phyto-chemicals.

It is my firm opinion that phytonutrients are an essential part of good health. The best way to obtain phytonutrients is to ingest the recommended daily intake of fruits and vegetables. This is two or three pieces of fruit and three to five servings of vegetables. There is no doubt from all of the medical studies that populations consuming these amounts of fruit and vegetables have much lower rates of heart disease and cancer. The unfortunate fact is that only 10 per cent of Western society ingests fruit and vegetables at this level. The answer is not to rush out and buy vitamin, mineral and trace metal supplements to avoid eating fruit and vegetables. You should obtain the freshest source of fruit and vegetables available.

It is timely to point out that during the past 25 years the concentration of vitamins, minerals and trace metals in fruit and vegetables has been reduced by around 30 per cent. Therefore, it is also my firm opinion that we gain added insurance from taking vitamin supplementation. The unfortunate problem, however, is knowing exactly what is the *best* supplement to take and at what dose you should be taking it. It is very important to realise that with vitamins, minerals and trace metals more is not always better. In fact, taken in excessive doses, these supplements can be toxic. That is why it is always better to obtain advice from a skilled health professional who has knowledge in this area.

Once you have obtained the advice and are confident your source of supplementation is high quality, combine your daily intake of fruit and vegetables with this high-quality supplement. You are then well on the way to Cell Factor nutrition.

PROTEINS

In the days of hunter–gathering, around 30 per cent of the diet came from protein. Most of this protein was from wild game, which is around 5 per cent fat. Most of that fat was unsaturated fatty acids, such as mono-unsaturated fats and essential fatty acids. The domesticated animals of our modern era, however, are around 30 per cent fat, and most of these fats are saturated fats. Our diets today are around 12 per cent protein, at a maximum, 15 per cent. In the days of our hunter–gatherer ancestor, the carbohydrate intake was around 45 per cent. All of those carbohydrates were natural carbohydrates from plant sources and not the refined carbohydrates we are consuming today.

Over the past 10 years there has been renewed interest in the high-protein/low-carbohyrate diets popularised by Dr Robert Atkins in the 1970s. Many of these diets recommend somewhere between 25 and 35 per cent of caloric intake in the form of proteins. This is certainly unnecessary and would be considered excessive. The Cell Factor diet is more 20 to 25 per cent protein, 45 per cent carbohydrate and 30 to 35 per cent fat, with most of those fats coming from essential fatty acids and monosaturated fats. Recent recommendations for a balanced diet from most conservative dietary associations or cardiologic associations suggest somewhere between 12 and 15 per cent protein, 55 and 60 per cent carbohydrate and 25 and 30 per cent fat. The questions we must ask ourselves are: where do proteins fit in with the other two macronutrients? and are all proteins created equal?

As I have stated, we need three macronutrients—fat, carbohydrates and protein—to drive all of the reactions within our cells. Carbohydrates, and in particular, glucose, are seen as the major fuel with fat being a secondary fuel but a vital aspect of membrane function. Proteins are, in reality, the backbone of most of the components that make up our body.

Amino acids are the building blocks for the protein. Amino acids contain carbon, hydrogen, oxygen and nitrogen, and some amino acids contain sulphur. When you think of protein and amino acids you think of muscle power and brain food. It does, however, extend further than this because proteins and their building blocks contribute to almost every basic bodily function. Proteins regulate and maintain the body—hormones, the balance of fluid within our body, blood clotting, immunity, vision and cell repair are all performed basically by proteins.

Proteins can be used as an energy source and this is usually around 4 calories per gram of protein. We basically need about 20 amino acids for our body to function normally. Nine of these are essential and 11 are non-essential.

The most complete form of protein containing *all* of the essential amino acids is animal protein. The reason for this is that animals have a similar muscle structure to humans. Plant proteins, which do not have a similar structure to human muscle, do not have the complete sequence of essential amino acids; therefore, they are considered lower-quality proteins. But, by combining different types of plant proteins you can still obtain all of the nine essential amino acids. (Interestingly, the only plant protein that does have the complete complement of essential amino acids is the soy bean.)

When a whole group of amino acids is joined together, depending on the amount of amino acids, they either become a peptide molecule, which contains less than 100 amino acids, or a protein, which has more than 100 amino acids. But, how are proteins formed in the first place?

Classification of amino acids

Essential (indispensable) amino acids	Non-essential (dispensable) amino acids
Histicline	Alanine
Isoleucine[*]	Arginine
Leucine[*]	Asparagine
Lysine	Aspartic acid
Methionine	Cycteine[†]
Phenylalanine	(Cystine)
Threonine	Glutamic acid
Tryptophan	Glutamine
Valine[*]	Glycine
	Proline
	Serine
	Tyrosine[†]

[*] A branched-chain amino acid.
[†] These amino acids are also classed as semi-essential. This means they must be made from essential amino acids if insufficient amounts are eaten. When that occurs, the body's supply of certain essential amino acids is depleted. Researchers now suggest that some other non-essential amino acids assume a more essential status when the body cannot readily generate them. This occurs during some illnesses. Glutamine may assume an essential status in traumatic injury, especially in the period after intestinal surgery, and arginine is essential for infants and children.

DNA pretty much contains the blueprint for all the proteins our body needs and is continually sending out its wonderful message to the cell to instruct it to make more protein. Our cells are constantly turning over protein by breaking down the existing protein and synthesising new proteins. The waste product of all of this protein turnover is urea. All of this metabolism takes place in the liver, which sends the urea to the kidneys, which dutifully sends it to our bladder and . . . you know the story from there. During any particular day the average adult breaks down around 30 grams of protein and recycles the amino acids. The average 70-kilogram man requires somewhere between 50 and 70 grams of protein a day for normal metabolism.

The function of proteins

Around 50 per cent of the protein in the body is involved in maintaining structure. Collagen and the muscle proteins make up this bulk. Another vital protein is haemoglobin, which transports oxygen around the body. Blood clotting, transport proteins, cholesterol-carrying proteins, enzymes and immune systems are also vital parts of body function. Hormones are commonly protein-based, although the steroid hormones, such as those used in reproduction, come mainly from fat.

Homeostasis is basically the balance in the body—the balance of fluid or the balance of pH or acid-base. Proteins sit on the membranes and regulate the flow of salt and potassium in and out of cells, along with many other chemicals, such as glucose, to assist balance. If you fast for too long and do not take in carbohydrates, your body will start making glucose from the amino acids in the proteins that have been broken down during normal day-to-day metabolism.

Protein foods

FISH

Over the past 10 to 15 years there has been a resurgence in fish eating. With our increasing concentration on lifestyle and health, many more people are eating fish not just for the taste, but also for the health benefits. We are constantly being reminded of the good, healthy oils and fats in fish. It is the wonderful Omega-3s that provide us with much of the benefit from consuming fish regularly, but we should also not dismiss fish as an excellent source of protein.

A standard serving of fish, which is usually 3 to 3.5 ounces, yields somewhere between 20 and 30 grams of protein. This is with little or no saturated fat. Compare this to the equivalent size of beef, with a saturated fat content anywhere between 4 and 10 grams, depending on whether the beef is lean or regular. So, for the equivalent amount of protein, fish is obviously the healthier choice than beef.

At this point, however, I must reiterate my comments that I do not believe that saturated fat is anywhere near as bad for you as trans fatty acids. Although saturated fat can increase cholesterol levels, it does not have the same effect on the membranes as trans fatty acids. My strong advice is that we enjoy two or three pieces of fish a week as part of our normal diet. The health benefits, both from the fat and protein viewpoints, are enormous.

EGGS

The much-maligned egg has been given a bad time over the years. The egg does have a fair bit of cholesterol (around 200 milligrams per egg), but one egg is only around 75 calories. It is an excellent source of protein with around 6 grams of protein per egg, negligible carbohydrate and 5 grams of fat, including a good proportion of essential fatty acids and mono-unsaturated fat. We have been told to have only one or two eggs a week but I would encourage you to eat them because of their protein and essential fatty acid content, especially the Omega-3 supplemented eggs.

NUTS

When the divine designer sat down to organise the physical dimension, He (or She) basically gave us all the means for a good healthy existence from our natural environment. One of the greatest packages nature designed was the group of foods called nuts. I have already stressed the importance of nuts in terms of their good fat content, but I have not as yet touched on the protein content of nuts.

Nuts are particularly high in an amino acid known as L-arginine. Why is L-arginine important? If I asked you a Trivial Pursuit question, 'What is the biggest organ in the body?', many people would say, 'the liver', 'the heart', 'the lungs' or 'the brain'. But the correct answer is 'the skin'. Yes, 'that wonderful covering that gives dermatologists their Mercedes' is the answer if you are playing Trivial Pursuit. It is, however, wrong. The correct answer is 'the endothelium', which is the single layer of cells that lines every blood vessel in the body. To parody a ridiculous analogy, if you took out the endothelium and laid it on a flat surface, it would probably be equal to three or four football fields.

The endothelium is the largest organ in the body. It is only a single layer of cells but is an actively functioning unit. When you are forced into a position of terror and you need to either defend yourself or run, signals are sent to the endothelium through your fear–fight–flight system to release a substance known as nitric oxide. The science buffs will remember that nitric acid was awarded the prestigious Molecule of the Year in 1992.

Nitric oxide is basically a ubiquitous vaso-dilating factor—it opens up your blood vessels to their maximum capacity delivering high-quality, high-flow blood to the muscles. This is a pretty good thing to have when you are trying to defend yourself or run away, as blood flow to the muscles delivers acute nutrients to the muscles and, therefore, improves muscle strength and function. During times of terror, your heart also has an increased blood flow and works around five times harder than it does at rest—again, all good things to have when you are trying to survive some sort of attack on your person.

The last thing you need, however, when you are in a deep sleep in the middle of the night, is torrential blood flow to your muscles, so your body releases the opposing chemical, known as endothelin to restore your blood flow and heart pounding to normal levels.

Nitric oxide comes from L-arginine in our food. It is, therefore, important that we take in good sources of L-arginine every day so we can nourish our endothelium, to allow us to produce nitric oxide when we need it to. I also believe that this is one of the reasons we see the 50 per cent reduction in heart disease in people who have 10 to 15 nuts a day. Walnuts, almonds and macadamias not only contain wonderful fats that protect us, but also contain high proportions of L-arginine, which improves blood flow to our heart and muscles and maintains good endothelial function. It is vital for us to concentrate on the health of our endothelium as initially it is damage to the endothelium that allows fat to escape across the damaged cells into the sub-endothelial space and set up fatty plaques, which is, of course, the precursor to atherosclerosis and heart disease.

Researchers have found that meals high in processed fats and carbohydrates can acutely affect the function of the endothelium by around 50 per cent over a few hours after the meal. Researchers have also found significant impairment in endothelial function in teenagers who smoke.

There are so many ways to damage your endothelium, but there are also so many ways to ensure the health of your endothelium. Surely it's not that difficult to swallow 10 to 15 nuts per day. That's one of the reasons I stress the need for a good breakfast.

Starting the day with a good L-arginine hit is a superb way to nourish your endothelium. It is important to realise that it is the blood vessels that are the delivery system for all nutrients—if the blood vessels are not functioning properly, then the nutrients are not delivered properly to the cell, and thus a breakdown in Cell Factor nutrition.

L-arginine is not only found in nuts, but is also present in fish, garlic, lentils, alfalfa and onions. L-arginine is also found in very high concentrations in legumes (all members of the bean family).

MUSHROOMS
Mushrooms are a reasonable source of protein and have been called 'the vegetable version of meat' by some experts. They contain a significant amount of B-group vitamins and iron, and around a gram of protein per 50-gram serve. The very popular shiitake mushroom has no protein and no fibre, but unlike the common mushroom, it has 10 grams of carbohydrate. Anyone who enjoys mushrooms regularly will be well aware of the after effects on the gastrointestinal tract. Mushrooms have been long used in Eastern medicine for their healing properties. The shiitake mushroom and the more recently described ganoderma mushrooms are alleged to have a possible anti-tumour affect. Mushrooms make an excellent accompaniment to many meals and I would strongly suggest using these wonderful substances liberally.

MEAT
For all its negative press, meat (including red meat) is still a wonderful source of protein. Although I am not suggesting that we should be having steak tonight, chops tomorrow night, baked dinner the next night, followed by sausages and so on as our regular diet, I believe their health detriments have been overdone. If you look at the Seven Countries Study, the people with the lowest rates of heart disease in this study were the people of Crete. They consumed red meat on two occasions a

month. The Okinawans from Japan have the largest groups of centenarians in the world and pork is part of their regular diet.

Chicken: Many people fear chicken more than they do other meats. There has been a health scare that chickens are being fed a whole host of chemicals, including antibotics and steroids, to prepare them for our consumption. What is the truth? The health authorities and leaders of these industries reassure us this is not the case. Others inform us that we're all being conned by these organisations, who put profits over people.

I can give you no clear answer along these lines. I would, however, like to make one observation: when I look at this generation of children, teenagers and young adults and compare them to my generation, I believe it is obvious that they are all taller and bigger. If you watch film clips of sporting events, concerts or even movies from the '60s and '70s, you see a whole host of relatively scrawny athletes, performers, actors, etc. Today's young athletes, performers and actors are much bigger, bulkier and taller. This may be purely due to the improved training methods and, possibly in some cases, the illegal use of anabolic steroids, or it could also be due to the additives of steroid hormones, antibiotics and other chemicals to the animals we are consuming.

Do I eat chicken? Yes. Once or twice a month. It is certainly very difficult in this situation to give you the right answers but, as I said, I'd be more concerned about a processed packaged food that had been sitting on the shelf for a few months and the effects that it may have on my body than something I would buy in a butcher's shop or chicken shop and eat that day or cook within the next few days.

Turkey: Turkey is an excellent source of low-fat, high-protein food. I would strongly endorse the regular consumption of turkey.

Game meats: The advantage of eating non-domesticated animals is the low-fat content of the food. Just like turkey, all forms of game meats, such as venison, have very low concentrations of fat. Domestic animals have around 30 per cent fat, whereas game meat is around 5 per cent.

In Australia, many restaurants are now offering kangaroo meat, emu and even crocodile. Again, all of these are excellent sources of protein and should be encouraged. Claims are emerging for the benefits of emu oil. This is not because of its protein content, but because emu oil is a rich source of essential fatty acids.

Soy: Soy beans actually belong to the pulse, or legume, family. Pulses or legumes are the edible seeds of certain plants. The protein content of pulses is around 25 per cent when raw, but drops to around 6 to 8 per cent after cooking. This particular protein is a rich source of the amino acids L-arginine and L-lysine. The benefits of soy beans and their related food products are said to be legion. These benefits do not just come from the protein component, however.

Soy beans offer numerous benefits, including the complete mix of amino acids compared with animal protein. Soy beans are also significantly high in fat, being around 40 per cent of the total caloric content, with the main fat being the Omega-6 fatty acid linolenic acid. There is also a significant amount of alpha-linolenic acid, i.e. Omega-3 fatty acids. Soy beans are also a rich source of a group of phyto-chemicals known as isoflavones and also a reasonable source of calcium.

Around 25 grams of soy protein per day (which is the equivalent of consuming around 250 millilitres of soy milk a day) could be expected to reduce cholesterol levels by around 5 per cent. When compared to the very powerful cholesterol-lowering drugs, statins, this is not particularly strong but still has some benefit. As I continue to state throughout this book, it is not purely the effect on cholesterol that is important, and there has been much work to show that the other components of soy bean, such as the isoflavones, can have an effect on other aspects of blood-vessel function that are important in helping to prevent heart disease.

Professor David Jenkins from the University of Toronto has completed a recent study using the 'Portfolio Diet'. This diet comprised five components:

1. Soy protein, 40 grams per day—soy milk, yoghurt and tofu.
2. Plant sterol cholesterol-lowering margarine.

3. Oat-based breakfast.
4. Almonds—10 to 15 raw almonds per day.
5. Increasing the consumption of fruit and vegetables.

The study participants demonstrated a 35 per cent reduction in LDL (bad) cholesterol, comparable to the effects of a strong cholesterol-lowering drug such as a statin.

The isoflavones in soy have been shown to have an effect on different types of common cancers. These isoflavones have specific effects against breast and prostate tumours, but large studies are still needed to confirm the association. In studies of large communities, it has been suggested that people who consume between one and two servings of soy products a day have around a 70 per cent reduction in prostate cancer.

Soy protein has been specifically shown to reduce the calcium loss from bones that is seen in people on a high-protein diet. Therefore, it may also be wise to consume two or three soy meals a week in the form of tofu and soy burgers, and to use soy milk.

Proteins—the downside

With the shift in emphasis away from low fat/high carbohydrate, there has been a plethora of books supporting the high-protein/low-carbohydrate way of eating. Therefore, the obvious question is: do high-protein diets have any possible harm? And if there is harm, is the harm directly related to the protein intake or possibly due to the foods that you are *not* consuming?

High protein often means high fat. Although I have somewhat diminished the problems with consuming a diet that is high in saturated fats, I am still not dismissing the fact that there is a contribution from high-saturated fat diets and, therefore, serum cholesterol with its relationship to cardiovascular disease. As a cardiologist, I treat people every day with cholesterol problems and would not be foolish enough to dismiss this as a factor. Many of the high-protein diets do not highlight the problems from excessive amounts of meat and the definite association between excessive animal protein intake and coronary heart disease.

The Adventist Health Study, which has followed 36 000 Adventists for well over 10 years, showed that this select group had longevity well above the average American and that their rates of heart disease were much lower. Adventists tend to be vegetarians, heavy consumers of nuts and legumes, non-smokers, non-drinkers, thinner and regular exercisers. The study demonstrated the independent benefit of consuming nuts as a replacement for meat. It has also shown the increase in bowel cancer in people who were meat-eating, non–fibre-consuming, overweight human beings, and it is difficult to decide which of these factors was the most important.

It is my opinion that, as with most things in life, the factors relating to disease are multi-factorial. People who are heavy meat-eaters tend to eat less fruit and vegetables and, therefore, have less fibre. They also tend to be more overweight. There are certainly much higher rates of bowel cancer in this group. One of the other possible reasons is that particularly well-done steak has a significant amount of altered chemicals in the form of heterocyclic amines and these have been associated with high rates of tumour growth.

Excessive amounts of *anything* may cause trouble. Excessive protein intake can increase the calcium loss from bone and, therefore, promote the development of osteoporosis. Increasing calcium in the urine also contributes to the development of kidney stones.

High-protein diets alone have also shown, regardless of the calcium content, to cause a slight deterioration in kidney function. The recommended daily allowance for protein is around 10 per cent. Once diets are up to the 20 to 30 per cent range in people with other underlying diseases, such as diabetes or known chronic kidney disease, they will accelerate their disease on a high-protein diet. All of these facts highlight to me the importance of regular medical check-ups. A competent doctor is the best person to assess your general state of health. A normal creatinine, which is a good indicator of your overall kidney function, along with a simple urinalysis looking for protein, blood and glucose, is a very easy way to determine the health of your kidneys. Even something as simple as a regular check of your blood pressure can be most beneficial.

Proponents of high-protein diets do tend to suggest a reduction in fruit and vegetables, downplaying the benefits of these foods. They also criticise the natural sugar content of fruits and suggest that fruits contribute to the carbohydrate burden. By eliminating significant amounts of fruits and vegetables from our diet we markedly reduce our fibre content, not to mention all of the wonderful phyto-chemicals which are vital for good health.

One of my friends decided a few years back to start the Atkins high-protein/low-carbohydrate diet. Within two months, after a considerable amount of weight loss, my friend had developed acute haemorrhoids because of his reduction in fibre content and was soon in a hospital for a haemorrhoid operation.

There has been much hype and much misinformation, however, surrounding high-protein/low-carbohydrate diets. Dr Robert Atkins himself, now in his seventies, recently suffered a cardiac arrest. Many of his critics came right out and said, 'You see, his diet doesn't work.' To put Dr Atkins' cardiac arrest into perspective, for the past few years he has been suffering from a condition known as dilated cardiomyopathy, which is usually due to a virus attack on the heart muscle and has nothing to do with fat build-up in the arteries. Following Atkins' cardiac arrest and successful resuscitation, he underwent a coronary angiogram, which showed his arteries were absolutely clean. Not bad for a septuagenarian! This is just an anecdote and it does not prove any true safety from the high-protein/low-carbohydrate diet, but it does reinforce my point that each individual is different. Some will have lousy genetics that will require more intensive therapy, and others will have excellent genetics and may respond well to one particular type of diet.

HOMOCYSTEINE

Case study: George—George was in his seventies and had had by-pass surgery on three occasions, the first at the age of 50. Unfortunately, by the time he was referred to me, he had damaged a significant part of his heart muscle and was suffering what is known as 'congestive heart failure'. After my initial assessment with George, I asked him, 'Why do you have heart disease?'

George was bemused by this question as he had certainly never been asked before. He replied, 'I don't know. No-one has ever really told me.'

Personally, if I had any sort of heart disease I'd like to know why and what I could do to prevent it. When I looked at George's cholesterol it was normal, his blood pressure was normal and he had never smoked. It was obvious, however, was that he had had particularly vicious heart disease from his early fifties. I organised some fasting blood tests and was not shocked to find his homocysteine level in his blood was 48—the normal range being less than 10 micromoles per litre.

I started George on high doses of folic acid, B12 and B6, and within a few months his homocysteine level had dropped to around 15. Unfortunately, this was too late to reverse his heart disease, but with good therapy he still maintains a reasonable quality of life and hopefully his underlying disease is not progressing now that he is on specific treatment for the original cause.

One of the essential amino acids, methionine, which is commonly in high proportion in animal proteins, can readily be metabolised to homocysteine, which is a toxic amino acid that damages the endothelial lining of blood vessels, making your platelets stickier than normal and can also promote fat build-up in the lining of your arteries. These, of course, are three particularly nasty things that you don't want happening anywhere near your body. If you assess anyone below the age of 55 who has either had a heart attack, stroke or peripheral vascular disease (blockages in the arteries in the legs), around 30 to 40 per cent have levels of homocysteine levels above 10 micromoles per litre. If these levels are above 20 micromoles per litre, I would routinely measure the B12 and folic acid level, which may indicate, rarely, a lack of folic acid in the diet, malabsorption of folic acid or, more commonly, pernicious anaemia. Chronic kidney disease is also commonly associated with high homocysteine levels.

The link between high homocysteine levels and atherosclerosis is now well established. There is also no doubt that treatment with folic acid, B12 and B6 will reduce homocysteine levels back to normal in most cases. What has not been firmly established is if treating people with high homocysteine levels with these three combinations of vitamins will reduce the risk of vascular disease in those people with initially high homocysteine levels.

It is my opinion (not shared by many of my colleagues) that a fasting homocysteine test should be a routine test when screening someone for coronary artery disease. One group from the Minneapolis Heart Institute studied folic acid levels and homocysteine among people below the age of 55. They found a significant association between low folic acid levels and a high homocysteine, and, not surprisingly, in those people who did not supplement with a multi-vitamin containing folic acid, they found around one in five had evidence of a folic acid deficiency. Also, surprisingly, the same number had evidence of a riboflavin deficiency. (Riboflavin is also known as Vitamin B2, and a lack of riboflavin contributes to a high homocysteine level.)

Studies such as these certainly fly in the face of conventional wisdom that suggests we obtain all of the nutrients we need from our foods. If this is the case, why are we finding such a high proportion of people who are deficient in simple, natural chemicals such as riboflavin and folic acid? The answer is twofold: first, only around 10 per cent of people are ingesting the recommended daily intake of fruits and vegetables; secondly, the quality of our food is much less than it was, say 30 to 50 years ago.

Another interesting aspect of homocysteine metabolism is the association with Alzheimer's disease. An epidemiologist from the University of Kentucky has studied extensively the post-mortem brains of a group of Roman Catholic nuns. They showed a clear link between Alzheimer's and low levels of folic acid. This is very exciting as the low folic acid–high homocysteine connection is something that is very easily overcome. Encouraging the consumption of leafy, green vegetables and the daily ingestion of a multi-vitamin table with at least 400 micrograms of folic acid may help in preventing the carnage from not only

Alzheimer's disease, but also heart disease, stroke, cancer and, of course, birth defects.

Protein-based foods are a vital part of our normal diet. Animal proteins are a first-class source, but if you have made the life decision to become a vegetarian, by combining different types of vegetables you can still obtain first-class protein.

Although I do not subscribe to the high-protein/low-carbohydrate theories of some nutrition experts, I do believe we have focused too much on dietary carbohydrate and not enough on protein. As with all my suggestions, it is important to aim for the middle path of moderation. The over-ingestion of any particular foodstuff—whether it be protein, fat or carbohydrate—will in most cases, predispose one to harm.

So the next time you sit down to enjoy eggs benedict, I wouldn't be feeling that guilty—in fact, you're probably doing your body some good.

MINERALS

When we think of minerals, we think of some form of rock. Minerals are, however, a vital component of every reaction in our body. Minerals are present in almost all food and, without a constant supply of minerals, we would rapidly be making our way either up to the Pearly Gates or down to the fiery basement, which, incidentally, has no toilets. Yes, hell is damnation without relief. Our bodies are made from the same building blocks as all other life forms, which makes it much easier for nature to distribute. Our micronutrients are, of course, vitamins, minerals and trace metals. The mineral and trace metal story is very interesting.

If you believe the conservative nutritional world, we derive all of the minerals and trace metals we need from a healthy diet. If this is the case, why are many people in Western society succumbing to severe mineral deficiencies? The most common manifestation here is, of course, osteoporosis. If, on the other hand, you believe the makers of magical mineral supplements, there is now a confusing array of organic minerals including chelated minerals and colloidal minerals, and only their particular brand is of any value—swallowing the opposition's brand is tantamount to committing a rather rapid suicide.

A simple principle applies here: ingestion of any mineral supplement should take the form of as natural a source as possible. The best sources of minerals are fruits, vegetables, seeds, nuts and grains. Of course, in the case of calcium, dairy products are an essential source.

Unfortunately, one of the startling facts to emerge from the nutritional world over the past 10 years or so is that 25 per cent of our total calories now come from sugar and around 35 per cent from fat (and much of this synthetic, processed sugar and fat). Thus over 50 per cent of our calories come from foods with very poor nutritional value. The vitamin, mineral and trace metal content of these foods is very limited. With less than 10 per cent of people consuming the recommended five or more daily servings of fruit and vegetables, what can you expect in regard to mineral and trace metal deficiencies?

Calcium

Well over 90 per cent of the calcium in our body exists in our bones and teeth. Calcium is not only important in these areas, but also for almost every reaction in the bloodstream and reactions across most of the membranes in the body.

Calcium, for example, is laid down in arteries as a healing response to the build-up of fat. When you develop atherosclerosis, one of the first changes is fatty plaques forming in the wall of the arteries. As these fatty plaques are very friable and can break down, the body responds to this by delivering calcium to the site, to try to act as a scaffold to strengthen the plaque. This strengthening reduces the ability of the plaque to rupture and, therefore, reduces the ability of the plaque to cause significant problems, such as heart attack or sudden cardiac death if the plaques are in the coronary arteries. Many older people have deposited so much calcium in their arteries that it is unusual for them to suffer a heart attack as a consequence of a plaque rupture.

Calcium is also a vital part of the clotting cascade. Without calcium, clots cannot form. A reduced amount of calcium in the bloodstream can also cause significant muscle problems with twitching, cramps and muscle irritability. Interestingly, however, when we think of a calcium deficiency we usually think of osteoporosis. Unfortunately, it is not that straightforward.

Osteoporosis is not due to a pure calcium deficiency. It is, in fact, much more complex and more often due to a combination deficiency. To prevent osteoporosis we need calcium, magnesium, phosphorus, boron and other minerals and trace metals. One of the most bizarre aspects of managing osteoporosis is to start treating the condition once it has occurred. It is estimated that the average calcium intake in our diet is somewhere between 500 and 700 milligrams a day, which is around two-thirds of the recommended daily intake. I believe it is important to ingest somewhere between 1500 and 2500 milligrams of calcium a day, from both food and supplementation, from your early thirties.

The importance of ingesting a balanced mineral and trace metal dose on a daily basis is understated in our society. All of these minerals have effects way beyond their ability to maintain healthy bones.

Potassium
Potassium is the second major electrolyte after sodium (which is discussed in the chapter on high blood pressure). The body contains around 90 grams of sodium and most of this is outside the cells. There are around 140 grams of potassium in the body but most of this is inside the cells. There is a beautiful electrical balance between sodium and potassium which is vital for normal cellular function. If the body loses potassium on a long-term basis, through either kidney disease, diuretic therapy or fluid loss, the result is cardiac rhythm abnormalities, kidney problems and possibly a rise in blood pressure.

It is important to realise, however, that excessive amounts of potassium can also cause problems. The first sympton of excessive potassium in the bloodstream is death. It is important to run the potassium in the bloodstream somewhere between 3.5 and 5 millimoles per litre.

Magnesium
Closely aligned to potassium is magnesium. Magnesium is often forgotten by the medical profession. One of the most common causes of a low

potassium level is chronic diuretic therapy. Diuretics are often used for the treatment of high blood pressure or in people with heart failure. The diuretics deplete the body significantly of potassium, but also deplete the body of magnesium. Without a proper potassium–magnesium balance, there is a propensity to many problems, including cardiac rhythm disturbances, weakness and, many researchers would also argue, problems with the immune system and allergies, including asthma. Subtle deficiencies of potassium and magnesium are very common in people who die suddeny following a heart attack. Again, these facts support the argument that many people in society are subtly nutritionally deficient.

Copper

We usually associate copper with plumbing. Interestingly, those people who believe in copper deficiencies also believe in our own plumbing going bad, that is, a deficiency in copper can lead to weakness in the walls of blood vessels, which can lead to aneurysm formation and, at times, rupture. Some of the more outspoken members of the complementary medical society also believe copper deficiencies can contribute to grey hair and wrinkles. It is my impression that age is also a reasonable factor in this department as well.

Zinc

Zinc is a vital component of the body's internal or endogenous antioxidant brigade. There is a substance known as super oxide dismutase (SOD), which is one of the most important antioxidant systems in the body. Without zinc in proper amounts, SOD will not function correctly.

Zinc has also been used as a component of preventative treatments for colds and flu. There is also some work showing zinc to be beneficial for sexual dysfunction and prostate problems. The long-term scientific work on all of these aspects of mineral supplementation is certainly not solid but is showing great promise. Moderate doses of supplementation have not been shown to cause any problems, but with all my recommendations, it is important for you to discuss this with your doctor or competent health professional as, in rare cases, some of these supplements may cause harm.

Selenium

Selenium is growing in stature as an important trace metal. Many areas of the world have soil that is deficient in selenium. Selenium is a vital chemical for normal muscle function, and appropriate supplementation has been shown to reduce the risk of heart disease, cardiomyopathy and certain types of cancer.

Toxicity has been reported with intakes greater than 600 micrograms but somewhere between 50 and 100 micrograms a day is quite safe. Selenium can be found in brazil nuts, organ meats, seafoods, cereals and certain vegetables, such as broccoli and celery.

Mineral-containing foods

There is no doubt that low-fat milks, cheeses and yoghurts have high calcium content. For all the other minerals, five foods contain significant amounts of trace minerals:

- wholegrain foods, such as wholegrain bread and natural cereals
- nuts and legumes
- avocados
- leafy, green vegetables
- seafood.

ALCOHOL IN MODERATION

The English-born American comedian Henny Youngman once said, 'When I read about the evils of drinking alcohol I gave up reading.' Many medical societies throughout the Western world are very quick to warn us about the evils of alcohol consumption while encouraging their doctor members to join their wine clubs. There are so many double standards regarding the consumption of alcohol and it is important to put alcohol in its perspective.

From a purely social viewpoint, alcohol has a very prominent position. It is very unusual to attend a social function where alcohol is not served. Our pubs and clubs are full of people enjoying the ambiance but also enjoying a drink with each other. Many people enjoy alcohol with their evening meal and these days it is very common for many people to have a pre-dinner drink and a drink just before retiring (sleep, I mean—not from work).

The downside is, of course, the physical, emotional and social problems created by the consumption of alcohol. From a purely physical viewpoint, 80 per cent of drug-related deaths in our society are due to cigarette smoke and 17 per cent are due to alcohol. One in 20 people in our community carry receptors in their brain for alcohol addiction, and it is this 5 per cent of the community, who also have varying problems with alcohol consumption, that make up almost all of the mortality and morbidity statistics.

STANDARD ALCOHOLIC DRINK

One of the big problems in defining a standard alcoholic drink is the definition of a 'glass', 'bottle' or a 'nip'. Many people buy large glasses. A small bottle of beer is 375 millilitres, or the equivalent of a schooner. This is 15 grams of alcohol, not 10. Two bottles of what is known as a 'stubby' are, in fact, 30 grams of alcohol (10 grams above the recommended limit). When someone says they have two nips of scotch a day, I would strongly suspect these nips are not particularly measured and are much more generous than you would really imagine. The alleged 10 to 20 grams of alcohol from one or two nips of scotch are probably more in the 30–40 grams range. This may be one of the explanations why one of the studies showed a significant increase in heart disease and cancer in those people who are regular spirit drinkers. Here is what a standard measure is:

- One glass of wine (125 millilitres) equals 10 grams of alcohol.
- One glass of beer (285 millilitres) equals 10 grams of alcohol.
- One nip of spirit (50 millilitres) equals 10 grams of alcohol.

Basically, alcohol is a cellular poison and has the potential to damage every single cell in the body at toxic levels. There is a strong anti-alcohol lobby that firmly believes alcohol is an evil. Some of these philosophies have a religious basis. On the other hand, there is the powerful liquor industry who obviously has a strong vested interest in downplaying the damaging effects of alcohol and lauding the social and health benefits (if they truly exist).

Alcohol, also known as ethanol, can be considered a food primarily because it contributes energy to the diet (7 calories per gram). Alcohol is not digested in the gut but is rapidly absorbed into the cells of the gastrointestinal tract. The liver is the first port of call for alcohol, thus the long-known damaging effects on the liver from excessive ingestion.

Alcohol is produced by the fermentation of different types of foods. Fermentation occurs when particular types of bacteria act on the foods, producing alcohol, acid and carbon dioxide. Brewers' yeast is often used as one of the sources of an enzyme necessary to make alcohol. Beer is made from malted cereal grain. Wine comes from grapes, of course. Spirits come from any particular number of fruits and vegetables or grains, requiring a distillation process.

The ingestion of alcohol on an empty stomach leads to a marked increase in absorption, thus the warning not to drink without food in your stomach. This may be one of the reasons why wine seems to have more health benefits than the other alcohol group, because wine is often drunk slowly with a meal. The wine would become mixed in with the food and the absorption is more regulated.

The enzyme 'alcohol dehydrogenase' is the major enzyme used to break down alcohol. It occurs in the liver and in the lining of the stomach. Men actually break down around 30 per cent of the alcohol ingested, whereas women will only break down 10 per cent, due to their different physiology. Therefore, larger proportions of alcohol reach the liver in women than in men. For a man and a woman who are drinking the same amount of alcohol, it will certainly affect the woman more than the man.

When the rate of alcohol consumption is greater than the liver's ability to break down the alcohol, the blood alcohol level rises—which explains our degradation from a sensible, pleasant human being to an obnoxious pain in the butt.

Case study—I remember a strange little man who was drinking rather heavily one day and fell over in his backyard and damaged his elbow. When he arrived in the accident/emergency to have his elbow stitched he was at the pathetic stage, claiming to be worthless and of no use to anyone. We sewed his elbow and advised him to return the next day for an X-ray (as this was in the bad old days when X-rays were not available on a Sunday). A few hours later he returned even more drunk with a scalp wound and this time, completely obnoxious and aggressive, trying to punch the staff. I then invited two members of our police force to come and join the show. These two gentlemen, who were both well over 180 centimetres tall, came in to see this small man flinging punches. A good swift kick planted firmly in his backside calmed him down somewhat and then I was able to stitch up his scalp wound without much in the way of local anaesthetic. The two constables invited him back to 'their house' for the night and the next day he even rang to say he couldn't return for the X-ray of his elbow because he'd been detained elsewhere.

The effects of excessive alcohol consumption

One of the major effects of excessive alcohol ingestion is the problem of drink-driving. Many countries now have rigid drink-driving laws; some have even gone to the extreme of zero-alcohol levels in the blood—thus the concept of designated drivers. It is not just the driving of motor vehicles that presents a problem, but also the driving of any other equipment, such as a boat. Of course, there are very rigid laws regarding the piloting of aircraft and alcohol in the bloodstream.

Alcohol the night before can very much affect a person's performance in the workplace the next day. Excessive alcohol ingestion does not promote sleep—in fact, the normal sleep cycle is completely destroyed by excessive alcohol, often resulting in someone waking in the early hours of the morning and not being able to return to sleep. Even if the person does not fully wake during the night, their sleep patterns are so disrupted that they experience marked fatigue the next day. Although the effects of a hangover are related to the alcohol itself and its metabolites, some of the effects are also related to the exacerbation of sleep disorders, such as sleep apnoea. Therefore, one of the first methods of dealing with sleep apnoea in a typical sufferer is to minimise their daily alcohol consumption.

Many arguments and violent attacks (including domestic violence) are alcohol-related. Alcohol problems also increase the risk for suicide. As alcohol also strongly lessens people's inhibitions, excessive drinking increases the risk for sexually transmitted diseases and unwanted pregnancies. The more alcohol consumed, the more likely it is for the person to have multiple sexual partners, thus increasing the risk of all manner of diseases and, possibly, pregnancy.

In most cases, people with chronic alcohol problems eventually become alienated from their family and, at its greatest extreme, may become one of the ever-increasing number of homeless people in our society.

Many lives are lost on a yearly basis as a consequence of excessive alcohol consumption, not to mention the numerous social problems created. In any developed country, alcohol is consumed regularly by around half of the adult population. In the United States around 15 to 20 million people a year are declared alcoholics. There are usually around 100 000 deaths directly attributable to alcohol on an annual basis, costing the community billions of dollars. Around 20 to 30 per cent of people admitted to hospitals in the United States have alcohol-related problems.

Many common cancers have an association with excessive alcohol consumption. These include all the cancers of the upper gastrointestinal tract and particularly the oesophagus. Colorectal (bowel) cancers and liver cancer have also been associated with this. There is also a weak association between breast cancer risk and excessive alcohol consumption.

This risk of breast cancer is in women who ingest more than two glasses of alcohol a day—especially if they do not take folic acid. In the Nurses' Health Study, is was clearly shown that the ingestion of a multivitamin with 400 micrograms of folic acid each day abolished the risk from breast cancer with low-dose alcohol consumption. Some researchers claim that women with a combination of a strong family history of breast cancer, early onset menstruation and benign breast disease should avoid alcohol completely.

When we think of excessive alcohol consumption we usually think of liver damage, but it is not just the liver that is affected significantly by alcohol. Many different organs can be damaged in some way. Absolute toxic levels of alcohol consumption is anywhere above four standard drinks for a male and probably two standard drinks for a female. I am not suggesting that if you occasionally go above this level you will definitely develop some long-term toxic side effect, but many people ingest well above this level every day. Although it may take over 20 years for this to have consequences, it usually does have consequences.

Specific organ and tissue damage

THE LIVER

Being the first port of call for alcohol once it is absorbed, the liver is a very important metabolic site. The direct cellular poison, being alcohol, destroys the normal liver metabolic pathways and, therefore, as the liver is an important site for fat clearance, when it is damaged by alcohol one of the first changes is fat accumulation in the liver. Non–alcohol-related fatty liver is also a common occurrence in Western society (commonly associated with insulin resistance syndrome) but in any person who presents with a fatty liver, the first question is, 'How much do you drink?'

The liver has very strong regenerating properties and within a short period of time after the cessation of alcohol, the liver can return to normal. Chronic excessive ingestion of alcohol, however, will lead to a scarring process known as cirrhosis. This is the fourth most common cause of death in people between the ages of 25 and 65 years of age. Once a liver has become cirrhotic, it will not recover completely. In a cirrhotic liver, the veins draining into the liver increase in pressure, causing enlargement of the spleen and the veins around the lower end of the oesophagus, known as varices. Chronic alcoholics with this complication can often bleed from the varices and, at times, may even die from this dreadful condition known as portal hypertension.

Case study: Jane—Jane was in her early thirties. She was one of the most addicted people I had ever met. She smoked 40 to 60 cigarettes a day, could not walk past a bottle shop without purchasing some cheap form of liquor and was an ex–heroin addict. She was admitted under my care at the local hospital with an ulcer on her lower leg that would not heal. After a few days of bed rest, antibiotics and dressing to the ulcer and, most importantly, no drinking, the ulcer healed quite well. Within a few days of discharge she was back to her addictive habits and was constantly being admitted to hospital or attending my clinic with alcohol-related problems.

I had had numerous conversations with Jane regarding the issue of her alcohol consumption and on each occasion she reassured me she would not drink again. After several months of this behaviour, she was admitted to the hospital with a severe gastro-intestinal haemorrhage from bleeding oesophageal varices. She rapidly developed what is known as a liver coma. Despite appropriate treatment, Jane died a few days later, leaving two small children without a mother.

Excessive alcohol consumption can also cause acute alcoholic hepatitis, total liver failure and even alcohol-related diabetes.

THE BRAIN AND NERVOUS SYSTEM

Alcohol has a direct toxic effect on many aspects of brain function. This is especially so in people who have a severe alcohol problem and also eat poorly (which applies to many alcoholics). These people often have a thiamine (Vitamin B1) deficiency. The combination of the toxic effects of alcohol and the thiamine deficiency can contribute to a brain syndrome known as Wernicke's encephalopathy. In this condition, the sufferer has severe eye problems or Korsakoff's psychosis. They suffer severe loss of short-term memory. Thiamine is routinely given to these people with only partial benefit. By the time people have developed either of these syndromes, it is often too late to achieve total recovery in many cases.

Another severe brain and central nervous condition related to excessive alcohol consumption is peripheral neuropathy. Peripheral neuropathy is damage to the peripheral nerves. There is a loss of sensation in the hands and the feet which in many cases is permanent.

Even without these three distinct alcohol-related syndromes, many excessive drinkers can develop a dementia-like illness. When a CT scan of the brain is performed, there is a lot of space around the brain which normally should not be there.

THE HEART
Although we are often told of the benefits of low-dose alcohol consumption in regard to a reduction in cardiovascular disease, there is no doubt that excessive alcohol consumption may lead to significant cardiac problems. The most common alcohol-related cardiac problem is a condition known as atrial fibrillation. Atrial fibrillation is the most common cardiac rhythm abnormality.

The atria, which are the two lower pressure chambers at the top of the heart, are basically holding chambers. Their job is to deliver blood to the thicker pumping chambers—the ventricles. There is normally a smooth coordination between the atria and the ventricles based on pressure chambers within the heart. It is, however, quite hard work for these poor low-pressure chambers, the atria, to continually pump blood into the higher pressure ventricles all day and every day.

The electrical system, which starts at the top of the atria, on the right-hand side in an area called the sinus node, sends natural electrical wires through both of these chambers into the junction of the atria and ventricles, known as the AV junction. This holds up the impulses to allow the filling of the ventricles, then sends an impulse through the ventricles in specialised fibres to allow a smooth contraction of the ventricles. This system allows for an efficient pumping action, maintaining a good cardiac output throughout our bodies. The electrical system, however, is very sensitive to the effects of toxins. Whether this toxin is the poisons we are exposed to on a day-to-day basis, whether it is a virus, or whether it is the very common poison of alcohol, the electrical activity can be affected.

Most of us realise this after we've had a very strong cup of coffee or a few cans of cola-based drinks—our heart feels like it is jumping out of our chest. In atrial fibrillation the atria basically gives up the ghost and starts to quiver. This quivering, or fibrillation, then leads to disordered messages being sent to the ventricles and thus the ventricles, instead of beating somewhere between 60 and 90 beats per minute in a smooth, coordinated fashion, will beat all over the place. The consequence of this in the short-term is a significant reduction in cardiac output by the heart.

If the person's rhythm is not restored to normal, usually within around 48 hours, small clots can form in the lining of the atria. These clots can then kick off and go up to the head, causing strokes, or to other parts of the body, causing other forms of mischief. Atrial fibrillation occurs much more commonly as we get older, but I have still seen people in their twenties in atrial fibrillation, some of these being alcohol-related.

Many people who develop atrial fibrillation will have to begin lifelong warfarin to thin the blood and be on rhythm-controlling agents to keep in a normal rhythm. One of the major consequences of atrial fibrillation is the need for cardioversion. This is an electric shock through the chest (thankfully performed under a general anaesthetic), but as with all things medical, prevention is the better cure.

The common setting for atrial fibrillation is the middle-age male with borderline blood pressure problems who has a big night on Saturday and either wakes on Sunday morning or even Monday morning in atrial fibrillation. The combination of blood pressure and atrial fibrillation is quite potent in this setting. Any more than two standard drinks of alcohol a day has a strong tendency to elevate the blood pressure. The risk for stroke is also much higher in alcoholics related to or, at other times not related to, hypertension.

Another important issue is the effect on blood triglycerides. Excessive users of alcohol have much higher triglyceride levels compared with people who are light or non-drinkers. Alcohol also has the tendency to raise the blood sugar by a number of different mechanisms. The most serious consequence of alcohol-related heart damage is severe cardio-myopathy. The heart muscle under these circumstances cannot pump enough blood to meet the needs of the body.

THE GASTROINTESTINAL TRACT

The stomach and pancreas are often affected by excessive alcohol consumption. Alcohol can lead to a gastritis; in its most extreme form a person with alcoholic gastritis can have a significant gastrointestinal bleed. There is a higher incidence of peptic ulceration among alcohol consumers as well.

The pancreas can also be affected by excessive alcohol. Acute pancreatitis is a life-threatening condition associated with an acute alcoholic binge. If the pancreas goes into 'meltdown' from excessive alcohol, it may have disastrous long-term effects. Alcoholics who experience chronic pancreatitis develop severe recurrent abdominal pain and can often become addicted to narcotic analgesics as a consequence of the pain from the pancreatitis. The damage to the pancreas is one of the mechanisms of diabetes seen relatively commonly in alcoholics.

Ascites is the accumulation of fluid in the peritoneum. This is usually related to liver damage but can also be due to recurrent peritoneal infections. This is a common long-term complication of cirrhosis of the liver. Ascites leads to marked fluid swelling of the abdomen and is rather difficult to manage.

NUTRITION

One of the major complications of alcoholism is poor nutrition. Many alcoholics consume little food throughout the day and often this food is of very poor quality. Why waste good alcohol money on expensive food? Because of this, many alcoholics are deficient in a range of vitamins and minerals. These deficiencies also contribute significantly to many of the complications of chronic alcoholism.

One of the problems here is changing the motivation of the alcoholic to consider their total body health. This highlights the importance of support groups for alcoholics, such as Alcoholics Anonymous. Having the association with like-minded people probably gives alcoholics the strength to help them recover from their problems.

Malabsorption is a less common consequence of excessive alcohol consumption. Malabsorption means nutrients are not getting into the body from the gastrointestinal tract. This can result in severe diarrhoea and a condition known as steatorrhea, which is the production of fatty, foamy, greasy stools. This is the sort of bowel action that could induce permanent 'sinus damage' to the next unfortunate person who walked into the bathroom!

It would not be complete to discuss alcohol without mentioning the potential effects on an unborn child. One of the problems regarding foetal alcohol syndrome is that much of the damage occurs in the first 12 weeks of pregnancy. Often women are not aware they are pregnant, and one episode of binge drinking can induce this syndrome, as can regular consumption of four or more drinks per day. This is somewhat analogous to the situation of thalidomide, which had to be taken on a particular day post-conception to cause the phocomelia (marked reduction in growth of the limbs).

Probably the safest advice for women considering pregnancy, or with established pregnancy, is not to drink at all. The usual manifestation of foetal alcohol syndrome is low birth-weight babies, facial deformities and mental retardation. There are six specific facial deformities, including a small head circumference, eye folds with a low nasal bridge, short nose and a small mid-face with a thin upper lip. These are classic features and it is not vital for all of these to be present to make the diagnosis of foetal alcohol syndrome.

A healthy mother produces a healthy baby. To prepare for your pregnancy, I believe it is important to prepare your body, preferably for three months before conception. Unfortunately, most people don't plan pregnancies to this level, but practising all the principles set out in this book will give your baby the best chance of being extremely healthy.

There are two other interesting problems related to alcohol consumption. Very rarely, people who consume only one or two glasses of alcohol can exhibit extremely violent behaviour. The other problem is a rare tumour of a small gland in the brain known as the pineal, which secretes melatonin, vital for the sleep–wake cycle. A tumour of this region can (very rarely) produce a syndrome known as alcohol-induced nymphomania.

Benefits of alcohol

After all this doom and gloom related to alcohol consumption, many of you are thinking, Why bother at all? The reason to bother is that most of us can enjoy alcohol in low doses and the evidence is now becoming overwhelming that low-dose ingestion of alcohol does afford some benefit. I must say, however, that the benefit is not enormous and for those of you who still have a reason, whether it be religious, social or lack of enjoyment of alcohol which prevents you from drinking, I would not suggest you force yourself to partake. This is all common-sense stuff.

When considering the beneficial effects of alcohol on the body it is important to ask yourself the following five questions:

1. Is *all* alcohol harmful?
2. Is there a safe dose?
3. Is any particular alcoholic beverage more beneficial than others?
4. If there is a benefit, why is it beneficial?
5. Why are so many of the studies and messages so conflicting?

IS *ALL* ALCOHOL HARMFUL?
I've demonstrated clearly in the preceding discussion the hazards of ingesting alcohol above four standard glasses per day. This evidence is overwhelming for any type of alcohol consumption and once you have achieved this ongoing level in your body most days of the week, eventually, in most cases, there will be substantial harm.

IS THERE A SAFE DOSE?
There have been multiple studies performed on the association between moderate alcohol consumption and coronary heart disease showing a consistent benefit from the consumption of around one to two drinks a day.

IS ANY PARTICULAR ALCOHOLIC BEVERAGE MORE BENEFICIAL THAN OTHERS?
The totality of evidence from 60 prospective studies shows an across-the-board benefit from all types of alcohol consumed at low dose. The studies

that have considered alcohol in general usually show around a 20 to 30 per cent reduction in cardiovascular disease from all forms of alcohol.

A number of years ago a study I will loosely call the Rabbit Alcohol Study took six groups of rabbits and fed them a diet high in processed fats and carbohydrates, inducing severe atherosclerotic disease over a three-month period. Each group was fed a different fluid and the percentage of atherosclerosis was determined.

The first group of rabbits was given water as their fluid and 100 per cent developed severe atherosclerosis. Group number two was given beer, and again 100 per cent developed atherosclerosis. Group number three was given whisky but the degree of atherosclerosis now dropped to 83 per cent. When the supplemental fluid was pure alcohol (and I wouldn't suggest this as a beverage), only 75 per cent of the rabbits had developed atherosclerosis. With white wine, only 69 per cent had developed atherosclerosis. The atherosclerosis rate for the rabbits given red wine as their major fluid was down to 40 per cent.

Was this something that was peculiar to the furry little rodents, or did it also occur in us human beings? The answer to this came from two major studies, one performed in Denmark on 13 000 people over 12 years and the other in France studying 36 000 people over the same period. The results were quite astounding. In the Copenhagen Heart Study, the consumption of one to two beers a day showed no benefit or detriment over the teetotallers. The consumption of two or three nips of spirits a day, however, showed a 30 per cent increase in heart disease and cancer.

My explanation for this is people's inability to judge the size of their nips. I suspect the person who says they are having two or three nips a day, if measured properly, would find they were probably having closer to four or five.

The most astounding evidence came from those people ingesting two or three glasses of red wine a day or, as in the French study, just two glasses a day. There was a 50 per cent reduction in heart disease and cancer.

IF THERE IS A BENEFIT, WHY IS IT BENEFICIAL?
I believe there are five good reasons why wine is more beneficial than the other forms of alcohol.

(i) Red wine has, in the skin of the red grape, a substance known as resveretrol. Resveretrol has antioxidant properties and also has a weak effect on lowering LDL cholesterol.

(ii) All alcohol has the propensity to raise HDL (good cholesterol) levels by somewhere between 6 and 10 per cent. Although this is only a weak benefit, it is certainly in the right direction.

(iii) Red wine does have a weak but definite blood-thinning property and, therefore, it reduces the ability for the blood to clot, thus reducing thrombosis.

(iv) Most importantly, red wine contains the three strongest dietary antioxidants known to man: quercetin, catechin and epicatechin. Taking 250 millilitres of red wine switches off 95 per cent of the free-radical attack on LDL, or bad, cholesterol. Why is red wine more beneficial than white wine? The reason is that there are 10 times the concentration of antioxidants in red wine compared with white wine.

(v) I believe the anxiety-relieving effects of coming home to the people you love and enjoying a lovely meal, slowly sipping two glasses of red wine, especially when consumed with the food, probably has enormous benefits over and above the science I have just mentioned. Again, I believe it gets back to the concept of balance.

Unfortunately, there is a downside to consuming red wine. A small proportion of the community will develop either asthma or an allergy related to the histamines in the red wine. There are also some unfortunate people who develop a 'red wine headache' or, even worse, severe migraines. If you are unlucky enough to fall into this category then you should avoid drinking red wine. For those of you who do not want to consume alcohol or have some sort of reaction to alcohol, there are a whole series of supplements, such as the grape-seed and pine-bark extracts or supplements with the red wine antioxidants such as quercetin, that can offer you a similar benefit.

Many people say to me, 'What about the ingestion of grape juice?' This, of course, contains the same antioxidants as red wine, but unfortunately, in grape juice the antioxidants are in a complex polymeric form, which means only 10 per cent of these are absorbed into the body following ingestion. When the wine is fermented the antioxidants are changed to a monomeric form which has an 80 to 90 per cent absorption rate.

There have been quite a few studies using de-alcoholised wine showing a similar benefit. Unfortunately, there have been no long-term studies and I suspect the small amount of alcohol probably does have some benefit.

A recent sub-study of the Male Professional Study showed doctors who consumed low-dose red wine had an 80 per cent reduction in sudden cardiac death.

WHY ARE SO MANY OF THE STUDIES AND MESSAGES SO CONFLICTING?

The reduction in cancer has certainly not been seen in any of the studies of alcohol consumption seen in the French study. If you examine the US data, there are numerous studies to suggest that there is only a 20 to, at most, 40 per cent reduction in cardiac events and no reduction in cancer rates. In some studies there is an increase in cancer rates.

My explanation for this is very clear. The US studies were performed, strangely enough, in the United States, where the diet is completely different from the European diet. The European diet, and in particular, the diet from France, contains a much greater proportion of antioxidants and much less processed and packaged foods. I therefore feel we should never look at one foodstuff (i.e. alcohol) in isolation, but consider the whole package of what travels into our gastrointestinal tract and therefore throughout the body.

I believe the data from the French and Danish studies is very solid but should be considered in its totality. I do not believe an agent, such as any form of alcohol, could override the harmful affects of a highly processed packaged diet that we see in countries such as the United States. Thus, the reason for the conflicting messages.

For those of you who enjoy your wine in moderation, every time you sit down to a meal you can slowly sip your wine knowing it is almost certainly offering you extra health benefits. There are some provisos to this message:

- You do not derive double the benefit from double the dose.
- You cannot save it all up for Friday or Saturday night. A binge of alcohol on one particular evening will knock your liver and the rest of your body around for quite a few days. The higher the dose, the longer the effect. By the time you have recovered from this excessive dose of alcohol it may be time for your next 'hit' on your body. A vicious cycle is formed.
- I am not trying to convince teetotallers to come out of the woodwork and start drinking alcohol. The reason for this message is to convince those of you who are drinking four or five glasses of beer a day or maybe three or four nips of spirit to pull this back to two glasses of alcohol a day, preferably red wine.
- It is the lifelong consumption through your adult years that will afford you this benefit. All of the studies have looked at long-term alcohol ingestion and not the acute benefit. There was, however, a recent study in *The Journal of the American Medical Association*, showing that people who were moderate drinkers in the year before their heart attack had a much lower death rate (around 20 to 30 per cent less) than those who did not drink at all.
- Most importantly, I have already mentioned that 5 per cent of the community have a strong tendency to alcoholism. If you have had an alcohol problem in the past, you should not see this message as justification to recommence alcohol. Alcoholics should go nowhere near alcohol on a lifelong basis.

Neutral foods

A QUESTION OF FAT?

It is extraordinary to me the misconceptions many people have regarding fat. If you polled most intelligent people in Western society regarding the greatest health risk in their diet, almost everyone would say, 'Fat.' There is, in fact, very little substance behind this misconception, which has been perpetrated over the last 40–50 years. As soon as someone gets a whiff of heart trouble, the first reaction is, 'Gee, I'll have to cut back on my fat intake.' I also hear other ridiculous comments such as, 'I won't eat prawns or other shellfish because it will raise my cholesterol.' With all this misinformation being thrown around from week to week, it's no wonder people are throwing their hands in the air and giving up in the dietary department. I have patients who swear blind they're ingesting a low-fat diet and proceed to tell me they regularly eat fish, use olive oil and eat avocado. These are three of the richest sources of fat in our society, but have also been shown to markedly reduce your risk for heart disease and cancer. We need to move away from this 'low-fat' concept because, firstly, it doesn't work; and secondly, there is now overwhelming medical evidence supporting the intense health benefits of all of these good fats.

The first misconception I would like to dismiss is that of dietary cholesterol. Foods that are high in cholesterol are:

- prawns and lobster, which contain around 110 milligrams of cholesterol per average serve
- eggs, each one contains 210 milligrams of cholesterol (exclusively in the yolk)
- liver (that is, paté) with around 400 milligrams of cholesterol per 85-gram serve
- kidney, containing 500 milligrams of cholesterol
- brains, with 2500 milligrams of cholesterol.

Firstly, there have been a number of studies showing that regular ingestion of eggs, prawns or lobster does not significantly raise the serum or blood cholesterol levels. Because of the complex metabolism of fat and cholesterol, once it has entered the body it is far too simplistic to think in terms of what goes in must manifest as what's happening in the bloodstream.

Dietary cholesterol really only accounts for a minimal contribution to the blood cholesterol level. It is my opinion that the protein content and the other nutrients contained in eggs, prawns and lobster override any unproven detriment from the cholesterol content of these foods.

As for the cholesterol content of liver, someone should inform the French that they should have much higher rates of heart disease than they do because of all the paté they are ingesting.

To take one component of one particular food and damn the entire food because of that component is blantantly ridiculous. Olive oil, for example, contains 14 per cent saturated fat. If indeed the saturated fat is causing any problems at all, it is certainly not being manifested in people who use olive oil.

It is quite interesting when you examine the cholesterol content of brains. Brains are really not what you'd consider a major component of most people's diet but it certainly makes the point—if brains contain such a high cholesterol content, then maybe there's something quite important about cholesterol. As I have stressed throughout this book, fats are a vital component of all our cellular mechanisms. Without good-quality fat, the membranes of our cells do not work; if the membranes of our cells do not work, the rest of our cells do not work. Cholesterol is particularly important in the brain, where it is a major component of the nerves and especially the covering of the nerves known as the myelin sheath. If the myelin sheath breaks down, the ability of your brain to perform its normal functions is markedly impaired.

Fats are divided into two categories, as follows:

1. Cholesterol: Cholesterol is the major sterol fat. A sterol has a par-ticular ring structure which is an important component of many body membranes, but also the basic building blocks of many of the body's hormones.
2. Triglycerides: Triglycerides make up 95 per cent of the body fat. Fat is stored in fat cells as triglycerides.

As your life progresses and the waistline rapidly expands to the point where you need to send out a search party to find your private parts, this enormous fat load is basically stored triglycerides. Triglycerides are a glycerol molecule with three lots (i.e. the 'tri') of fatty acid chains. The fatty acids can be the saturated fats, which, for those of you who love your science, means 'the chemical bonds between the carbons are all single connections and filled with hydrogen'—thus the word, 'saturated'. If they are not saturated then they are, strangely enough, unsaturated. The unsaturated fatty acids are either the mono-unsaturated fatty acids, which means there is one double carbon bond, or, if there is more than one double carbon bond, they're guess what . . . polyunsaturated.

The only reason this is important is the different properties of these fatty acids based on the degree of saturation or unsaturation of the sub-stances. The final type of fat is known as a phospholipid, the most famous one being lecithin. Simply put, this is a few fatty acids joined together with a phosphate molecule.

The real purpose of this chapter, however, is to discuss the real or perceived dangers of saturated fats. Firstly, there are quite a number of saturated fatty acids, most of which are not particularly operative in food. The fatty acids are divided into short-chain, medium-chain and long-chain fatty acids. Short-chain fatty acids have less than six carbons in their molecule and are usually liquid at room temperature. Dairy fats are a source of short-chain fatty acids. Medium-chain fatty acids contain between six and 10 carbons and are also liquid at room temperature. The best example of a medium-chain fatty acid is coconut oil.

It is the long-chain fatty acids, which contain more than 10 carbons, that are the ones that usually cause the mischief with your cholesterol. In fact, there are only three important fatty acids with between 12 and 16 carbons that appear to raise LDL cholesterol to any major degree. These include lauric acid (12 carbons), myristic acid (14 carbons) and palmitic acid (16 carbons). There is another long-chain fatty acid important in different types of food known as stearic acid, which has 18 carbons, but this does not appear to raise LDL cholesterol levels.

In most of these different oils and fats there are varying degrees of saturated fatty acids to make up the particular substance. For example, although coconut oil contains a significant proportion of medium-chain saturated fatty acids, there is also a large proportion of lauric acid, which tends to have a significant LDL cholesterol–raising property. Interestingly, red meats and chocolate contain a significant amount of palmitic and stearic acids. As I have stated, the stearic acid has little effect on cholesterol but the palmitic content of these foods has the potential of raising the cholesterol. Myristic acid is the major saturated fat found in dairy products.

The common sources of saturated fat in food are: meat (especially red meat), dairy products (especially milk, butter, cream and cream cheese), and certain types of oil—especially coconut oil, palm oil, lard, beef dripping, copha oil and chocolate.

Despite all of the hype regarding the ingestion of saturated fat, it really doesn't seem to translate into major health problems. In many ways, it is throwing out the baby with the bath water because many of the foods we ingest that have high proportions of saturated fat are prepared in hydrogenated oil (of which we are not usually informed), producing trans fatty acids. It is often difficult to separate the trans fatty acid content of a food from its saturated fatty acid content.

All we can do is look to the available science. When the Seven Countries Study was performed by Ancell Keys, there were only two heart attacks in the first five years in the particular village studied in Crete. One of these was the local town butcher. It is an important fact to stress that increasing your saturated fat intake by 5 per cent a day, which would probably equate to having an extra piece of steak every day, would increase your risk for a heart attack by around 17 per cent. Swallowing a muffin, a piece of cake or a few biscuits every day would increase your trans fatty acid intake by around 2 per cent, which equates to a 50–93 per cent increase in risk for a heart attack.

I am not suggesting you should see these statistics as a carte blanche to dedicate your life to the principles of carnivorism, but I also do not believe you should be sitting there with your razor blade poised over your radial artery every time you feel like a piece of steak.

These days we can also choose leaner meats, such as chicken and pork, if we want to enjoy a bit of animal protein.

Regarding dairy products, again, there are wonderful low-fat alternatives on the market that reduce exposure to saturated fat, but still provide us with an excellent source of calcium.

It is interesting that a nation such as France has a high cheese intake but has much less heart disease. I am not in any way suggesting cheese protects you against heart disease, but there is probably something in the fermentation process that does create some element of protection. Interestingly, the harder forms of cheese such as Parmesan and fetta cheese have reduced absorption in the gut, and also calcium in cheese products tends to bind fat, thus reducing the absorption of saturated fat within the cheese. I believe more work needs to be done in this area but again, I do not believe that it hurts to enjoy your cheese in moderation.

There is now recent work—the Coronary Artery Risk Development in Young Adults Study—that shows a significant benefit from the consumption of dairy products.This study was performed in Boston, Massachusetts, examining just over 3000 young adults between the ages of 18 and 30. The researchers monitored the participants for about

10 years, examining their intake of milk, butter, cream and cheeses. They found those who were overweight but consuming more than 35 servings of dairy products a week were 72 per cent less likely to develop insulin resistance syndrome (which is, of course, the major precursor to later-onset diabetes) than those who consumed less than 10 servings of dairy products per week.

Interestingly, this association was not seen in the participants with normal body weight. One of the proposed mechanisms from the researchers was that the fat in the dairy products might enhance the feeling of satiety (the feeling of fullness after ingesting a meal). This satiety may reduce cravings for the higher-carbohydrate foods that contribute to insulin resistance syndrome. The calcium, potassium and magnesium content in dairy products may also be of some benefit. This is further evidence that we should not pick one component of a particular food when other components may be causing significant benefit.

COMPLEX CARBOHYDRATES

Most of the modern recommendations for diets are to receive somewhere between 50 and 60 per cent of your energy intake from carbohydrates. There is no nutritionist out there who suggests a high intake of simple sugars, the major disagreement coming in the more complex, though still processed, carbohydrates.

The best forms of complex carbohydrates are, of course, fruit and vegetables. What makes fruit and vegetables so good for you is not the carbohydrate content, but all of the other phytonutrients contained within the food. It is still my firm belief that we are receiving far too much in the way of carbohydrates from other sources; if we have our designated three to five servings of vegetables each day and two or three pieces of fruit each day, we are receiving adequate amounts of carbohydrate.

In Western society we are very attuned to consuming bread. I still believe we consume far too much of the stuff but if you do wish to eat bread, I would strongly suggest you have wholegrain bread or even better, soy and linseed. I would also only suggest two or three slices of bread a day. Two slices of standard wholegrain bread contains somewhere between 25 and 30 grams of carbohydrate, with between 4 and 8 grams of fibre. I believe more than 15 grams of carbohydrate per serve is too much in the way of carbohydrate, so two slices of even grain bread is stretching the limit. If, however, you have a sudden energy craving, you're better off having either a slice of wholegrain or linseed bread or, preferably, fruit or nuts.

If you are eating rice, I strongly suggest brown rice over white and there are certainly some subtle differences in the different types of commercial rices available.

Some people believe what I have said about pasta is heresy. They immediately say, 'Just look at the Mediterraneans and their longevity. Pasta is one of their major foods.' We must also look to the Mediterranean lifestyle and its resultant low incidence of heart disease, cancer and diabetes. Those Mediterranean people who live a true village lifestyle have a large breakfast, with their lunchtime meal as the biggest meal of the day. They sleep after lunch and then toil in the fields in the afternoon burning off any food they may have ingested from the preceding meal. They have almost no evening meal, do not possess cars and generally suffer little stress. Mediterranean people who now live in cities do not live in this fashion, however. There is still a high rate of vascular disease, especially among many of the European populations that are heavy smokers, despite the fact that they are not particularly overweight.

If you choose to eat pasta I would strongly suggest you select wholegrain over commercial pastas. Again, should you avoid complex carbohydrates as well? Of course not, but it is important to remember that with all carbohydrates, no matter how complex they are, when you exclude the fibre component that is not absorbed, the remainder will end up eventually as sugar in your bloodstream. Whether this causes the acute glucose rise as seen with the high glycaemic index foods, or the slower glucose rise seen with the lower glycaemic index foods, it will still eventually end up as glucose. If you do not burn off this glucose, it becomes converted to fat. I believe it is this rather simple misconception regarding the alleged benefits of carbohydrate-laden food that has been one of the major factors in the generation of obesity and diabetes and all of its other consequences.

This is why I refer to saturated fat and complex carbohydrates as neutral foods. In many ways the foods containing significant amounts of saturated fat have been given too much bad press, while the foods containing the complex carbohydrates have been seen in too favourable a light. As with most things, I believe the answer is somewhere in the middle.

So, the next time you sit down to tuck into a beautiful piece of pepper steak, don't feel particularly guilty. Similarly, the next time you sit down to ingest a large bowl of wholegrain rice or pasta, I hope your halo doesn't choke you.

Exercise regularly

Every year, on a brisk Sunday morning towards the end of winter in Sydney, a race known as the City to Surf takes place. Thousands of Sydneysiders and many people from throughout the country and around the world travel to one of the main streets of the city to start the run (for quite a number of people, the walk) to Australia's most famous beach, Bondi. This 14-kilometre trek, which involves a section known as Heartbreak Hill, is not an easy undertaking. All manner of people take part in the race—from the very young, being pushed in strollers, to the very old, moving at varying degrees of speed.

Most years, there are casualties of some sort, occasionally fatal. The notion of such a public show of exercise raises many questions. What is the true value of exercise? Who should and shouldn't be exercising? How much exercise do we really need? Is exercise dangerous? What type of exercise is the best?

Oscar Wilde once said, 'Every time I think of exercise, I lie down till the feeling passes.' There are many people throughout the world who share Wilde's notion of physical exertion. There is, however, no doubt that exercise affords significant health benefits.

Before moving to a larger discussion about exercise, I believe it is important to consider a much-lost art in this society. I'm referring to a concept you may not have heard of before, a little thing called movement.

You have these things below your hips called legs. Unfortunately, many people feel that using their legs is an imposition on their existence. I don't know how many people I see using the escalators in large shopping centres when there's a perfectly good set of stairs right next to them. Think about it.

Many people wake up in the morning, drag themselves into the bathroom, empty their bladder, have a shower and drag themselves into the kitchen, where they may or may not have breakfast, but certainly have the obligatory cup of coffee. After a quick read of the newspaper, they hop in their car and drive to a parking spot next to the lift. It may be a few metres from the lift to their office. They sit at their desk all day, on the phone, answering emails and buzzing their assistant to get them their usual hits of coffee throughout the day. They may or may not leave the office for lunch. With the minimum of movement, they will return to their car at night, drive home, completely exhausted, swallow down a large meal laden with processed fat and carbohydrates, take up their position in front of the television with, of course, the remote control. When they have exhausted their desire to watch any more television, there's the long march into the bedroom. After six to eight hours of sleep, the entire merry-go-round starts again.

My friend Garry Egger, who started Gut-Busters® in Australia, feels it is this lack of movement that is the major factor in the obesity and diabetes epidemic we are witnessing in our society. For many years Garry has used a simple device known as a pedometer, which measures the steps taken in a day. One of the interesting features of Garry's research is that more than 10 000 steps creates weight loss, which seems like a hell of a lot, especially for the person I've just described. I have a number of clients who state they exercise for half an hour, four or five times a week, but the reality is that for 23½ hours a day they are basically immobile. The more immobile you are, the slower the metabolic rate. The slower your metabolic rate, the slower you metabolise fat. If you maintain your mobility throughout the day, you are always challenging your metabolism, and therefore your metabolism does not get the chance to switch off. The old adage 'Use it, or lose it' certainly applies here!

The five rules for movement are as follows:

1. Use the stairs and not the escalators or lifts, if possible. Of course, if you work on the twelfth floor, this is very difficult, but if you're only one or two floors up, develop the habit of taking the stairs.
2. Park further away from your destination. The first job I ever had was as a car park attendant at a local shopping centre. I must say, I found it a fascinating study in human behaviour. As soon as there was a whiff of a parking spot close to the front entrance, even the most fleet of foot among us would plant their car at the front of a long line of impatient shoppers and wait the obligatory five minutes for someone to unpack their shopping, rather than continue to the top of the parking area, which incidentally had a long down ramp for easy exit. The thought of having to walk the extra distance was a real anathema. I strongly advise aiming for a parking spot as far away from the entrance as you can get. These days, with the benefits of shopping trolleys, you get the added anaerobic exercise with your arms having to push the trolleys, along with the extra walk.
3. Walk/cycle to shops rather than drive. We are all creatures of habit. On Sunday nights my wife and I enjoy watching the latest video release. The video store happens to be about 2 kilometres away, so instead of driving down to pick up the video, we usually walk, and then do the same when returning it the following evening. This gives us a 4-kilometre, 30–40-minute walk on consecutive nights. There are many people, however, who jump in their cars to drive 500 metres to pick up a bottle of milk. If you are truly serious about maintaining good health and developing an exercise and movement habit, start to use your legs rather than your automobile.
4. Avoid the remote control. The more you sit in one place, using remote controls, the less you are keeping your metabolism moving. Once you have hit the age of 35, it certainly requires a major effort to get the limbs moving again after sitting in the one position for too long.

5. Don't stay glued to your desk. In this modern age where many jobs are desk-bound, we are certainly paying the price in the waistline stakes. Try not to sit in the one spot for too long when you're at work.

Apply all these principles as often as you can to maintain a constant burning of those calories.

Frequently asked questions

WHAT IS THE TRUE VALUE OF REGULAR EXERCISE AND MOVEMENT?

In medical parlance, there is a 30 per cent reduction in cardiovascular disease in people who are regular exercisers compared with non-exercisers. Exercise is, thus, a vital aspect of all cardiac rehabilitation programs. Cardiac disease aside for the moment, exercise has also been found to reduce the risk for many common cancers. Women who exercise regularly are far less likely to get breast cancer than those who do not. The reason for this is unclear, but may have something to do with the interplay between hormones, body weight and exercise. Incidence of pancreatic and prostate cancer have also been shown to be reduced in regular exercisers. For less serious, but equally as disabling, conditions such as asthma, there is also great benefit from exercise.

IS MORE BETTER?

Whether the studies are done on younger people or the elderly, it does seem there is a ceiling to the benefits derived from exercise.

Every day we see many seasoned exercisers pounding the streets, often with their finger on their carotid pulse, staring at their watch. Many wonder what on earth they are doing. For those who love numbers, 220 minus your age is the approximate figure for your predicted maximum heart rate. Once you have achieved around 60 to 70 per cent of your predicted maximum heart rate, this is when you start to burn fat and develop cardiovascular fitness. There is, however, a much simpler way of achieving this level than having to block off a major part of your cerebral circulation and check your pulse.

Rather than worrying about numbers, remember the two words, 'perceived exertion'. Perceived exertion is that feeling you have during exercise when you start to break into a slight sweat and feel a bit short of breath. It is actually a pleasant feeling. It usually occurs a few minutes into a light jog, or a few more minutes into a rather brisk walk. When you have achieved this level you are at around 60 to 70 per cent of your predicted maximum heart rate. It is my advice to maintain this feeling for around 20 minutes or so, four or five times a week. This is equal to around half an hour's exercise four or five times a week.

Forget about pulse monitors and checking your heart rate with your watch. Just listen to your body. Develop perceived exertion and maintain that feeling. Do you need to work yourself into a state of profuse sweating and gasping for breath? Of course you don't. There is no real benefit to the body's system in achieving this level of exercise compared with perceived exertion. In fact, the more you push your body beyond this limit, the more free radicals are released into your bloodstream from the excessive demand on your muscles.

Once the body's metabolism gets pushed beyond a level, the extra demand for oxygen in the tissues creates more free-radical by-products. When we are at rest, our cardiovascular system is really only working somewhere between 10 and 20 per cent of its maximum rate. When we push it to the maximum level, it has really only been designed as a form of protection to allow us to run or defend ourselves under times of threat. It is these extra demands on the body that predispose athletes to recurrent viral infections, and there are now scientifically designed antioxidant programs for high-performance athletes to reduce the free-radical damage. Although no scientific study has ever been performed along these lines, we often hear of high-performance athletes dying prematurely in their forties and fifties from either heart disease or cancer. I believe the reason for this is almost certainly related to the excessive free-radical load during the years of high-intensity exercise.

WEEKEND WARRIORS AND HIGH-INTENSITY EXERCISE

What about the 'weekend warriors' who play high-intensity sports, such as soccer, netball, basketball or squash? Should these games be avoided?

My answer to this is a definite, no. I must say, I am very biased—being one of them myself. Currently in my mid-forties I am still playing competition soccer. This is, of course, in a geriatric (over 35) competition, but it's still a reasonable level of soccer and induces a significant strain on our ageing bodies every weekend. I find this time a wonderful stress release, but certainly, it does take its toll on my lower limbs.

If you enjoy weekend sports, my suggestion is to try to continue these sports for as long as your body will allow, but to definitely consume higher levels of antioxidant dose vitamins and follow the cell-factor diet.

DR WALKER'S ANTIOXIDANT SUPPLEMENT RECOMMENDATION FOR SPORT PLAYERS ON THE DAY OF THE GAME

To be taken a few hours prior to participating:

- Vitamin E, 500–1000 international units.
- Vitamin C, 1 gram.
- Co-enzyme Q10, 50 milligrams.

If you are developing soreness in your knees and ankles and you are over the age of 35, it is worth considering regular glucosamine with chondroitin sulphate, along with 1000-milligram fish oil capsules twice daily (to be taken on a regular basis).

Squash still has a significant popularity throughout the world. Many authorities suggest people should not be playing squash beyond the age of 40. As this is a very intensive game requiring both aerobic and anaerobic activity, it does put quite a strain on the cardiovascular system.

Aerobic exercise is activity related to cardiovascular exercise. This includes exercise such as running, jogging, cycling or any of the other activities that get the heart pumping. Anaerobic exercise, however, is activity that requires the sustained actions of muscles, such as weight lifting, weight-resistance training or specific exercises that hold the muscles in one place.

Many people working in the field believe that anaerobic activity is just as beneficial for the cardiovascular system and weight loss as aerobic exercises. The advantage of performing more anaerobic exercise is the ability for body toning. Anaerobic exercise markedly improves muscle strength, especially in the upper limbs and abdominal muscles, and it is probably important for you to design a program that involves half an hour's aerobic activity a day and five to 10 minutes' anaerobic activity so that your body derives the benefits from both.

There are many regular gym attendees who achieve much more anaerobic activity than I have mentioned but the difficulty is deciding how much is best. If you decide to perform more anaerobic activity then you can probably cut down on your aerobic activity.

Back to squash . . .

Although I agree that squash is a very high-intensity activity, I do not believe it should be ruled out after the age of 40. I do think it is important for people who want to extend their bodies beyond the norm to have regular medical assessments over the age of 35. If you wish to play squash and have been given a clean bill of health from your doctor, there is no reason why you should not do so.

An ex–Australian prime minister, Sir William McMahon, played squash until he was 75 and died of an unrelated cause in his eighties. Many people over the age of 40 enjoy squash without any particular hazard or strain to their body. There was a study performed on 22 squash players who dropped dead while playing squash. Interestingly, 21 out of the 22 had either complained to a relative or a doctor of chest pain in the week preceding their death. The message here is not don't play squash; it is: if you have any concerning symptoms, such as chest pain, unexplained shortness of breath, dizziness, palpitations or unexplained fatigue, visit your doctor immediately. If you suffer any of these symptoms you should not play squash or perform any significant exercise until they have been thoroughly evaluated.

Case study: Jim Fixx—At the age of 32 Jim Fixx suffered a heart attack. At that stage, Jim was not particularly diligent in the way he handled his health. He was overweight, smoked, ate the wrong foods and had high cholesterol. So, he made the decision to completely reorganise his risk-factor profile and took up running.

He became world-renowed for his book *The Complete Book of Running*, and competed in many races, including marathons, over the next 17 years. At the age of 49 he developed chest pain. He mentioned this to his friends, who said, 'Jim, you are so fit you couldn't possibly have any further heart troubles!'

Jim suffered six weeks of intermittent chest pain and, on the morning of a race, complained of chest pains to one of the officials. Again, the comment was, 'Jim you're too fit to have any serious troubles.' Jim attempted to compete in the race but collapsed and died.

Was it the running that killed Jim Fixx? Of course not. It was the fact that no-one listened to his complaints of chest pain.

If someone with a background of atherosclerotic disease develops chest pain, it is highly likely they have ruptured a plaque within one of their arteries. Running at any level does not make you immune from progressive atherosclerosis and, although it is much better to be a regular exerciser than a non-exerciser, there is no guarantee that regular exercise will prevent any further vascular events.

IS EXERCISE AT ALL DANGEROUS?
There is no doubt that there are a few conditions—especially involving the cardiovascular system—that increase the risks during exercise. One of the major conditions is undiagnosed atherosclerotic disease. In people with significant atherosclerosis, even if it has not yet ruptured to cause a blockage, sudden exertion can precipitate a plaque rupture because of the extra stress on the cardiovascular system.

A study performed a number of years ago and published in the *New England Journal of Medicine* clearly demonstrated a significant increase in sudden death in people who were inactive but suddenly performed some form of exertion. For example, the middle-aged overweight man who has to run up the stairs to catch his train can put so much strain on his cardiovascular system that a plaque in the wall of his artieries can easily rupture. I too frequently hear the story of an inactive person who, when asked to perform a higher level of activity than normal, such as help his neighbour push his car when it wouldn't start, sustains a heart attack within a few days.

Unfortunately, unexpected significant exertion is just that—unexpected. In many cases it is difficult to avoid this exertion but it is important that you realise this may come at a price. If you have made a New Year's resolution or have been advised to start exercising, or have been given as a gift a subscription to a gym, and you have not exercised for a number of years and are over 35, it is my strong recommendation that you consider having some form of cardiovascular assessment prior to commencing exercise.

Another less common but very significant cardiac diagnosis, which should raise caution for anyone wanting to exercise, is one of hypertrophic cardiomyopathy, a genetic disorder that leads to excessive thickening of the wall of the heart muscle. It more commonly presents in young people, and people with this diagnosis are prone to sudden cardiac death, but especially during times of exertion or severe stress. I well remember during my training in cadiology a 23-year-old man, who knew he had hypertrophic cardiomyopathy, dying suddenly during a game of soccer. He was strongly advised not to exercise, but ignored this advice. Unfortunately, he arrived too late at the hospital and he could not be resuscitated.

Another tragic case was a professional triathlete in his twenties. In the running of one of his triathlons he collapsed towards the end of the race. He was resuscitated at the scene and, when assessed at a major teaching hospital, was found to have severe hypertrophic cardiomyopathy. An electrophysiology study was performed showing he had very disordered impulses travelling through his heart and required a pacemaker. He was advised not to compete in any more triathlons but, he informed the doctors, triathlons were his life. In his next triathlon he competed in, it was his death.

Anyone suffering severe hypertrophic cardiomyopathy should be strongly advised not to perform intense physical activity. Hypertrophic cardiomyopathy certainly contributes to a significant proportion of the sudden death in young people, especially in young athletes. The diagnosis can be confirmed by performing an electrocardiogram and an echocardiogram. The echocardiogram measures the thickness of the walls of the heart and appropriate treament can be commenced after the disgnosis is made.

There are numerous other causes for exercise-related cardiac problems but they are much less common than those already mentioned. If you suffer any cardiac symptoms or wish to start an exercise program over the age of 35 after having not exercised for a few years, I would strongly suggest you consider a full cardiovascular assessment prior to commencing any program.

WHAT TYPE OF EXERCISE IS THE BEST EXERCISE TO ACHIEVE YOUR AIMS?

Another important question to ask when considering exercise is probably the most obvious. First, you must decide *what* your aims are. If your aims are purely to achieve cardiovascular fitness and to keep your weight controlled, these are completely different from a desire to compete in the Boston Marathon. As I have stated, competing in any marathon or high-level sporting activity should not be seen as a way to achieve additional health benefits on top of my basic recommended exercise regimen. The best exercise is the exercise you will *continue* to do. For example, if you hate jogging, then don't jog. If you hate competition sports and appear to completely lack coordination, don't play competition sports. In reality, there is no ideal form of exercise, only the one you enjoy and will continue to do.

Exercise will not afford you any further benefit than for the time you spend exercising. What I mean by this comment is that within a few weeks of stopping the exercise you lose the health benefits. Therefore, any exercise program has to be a program for life, not a program for just a few months. Nor can you assume that your prior moderate-to-high level of exercise as a teenager and early adult will give you any protection whatsoever in your later years. Personally, I find exercising alone incredibly boring. I am not a jogger, nor do I find swimming laps of any interest whatsoever. Yet I do know many people who find jogging or swimming laps very meditative— it's their 'time alone' to contemplate aspects of their life.

One of my very good friends is a highly respected professor of medicine in one of Sydney's major teaching hospitals. He attends a gym three or four mornings a week and walks on the treadmill for half an hour. When I asked him what he does during this half an hour, apart from walk, he replied simply, 'Think.' Many people, when they have their regular morning or afternoon jog, or swim their numerous laps in a pool, develop a mediative rhythm and with the endorphins released during this exercise they become quite addicted to the activity.

My 'buzz' is competition sports and whether it be soccer, squash or tennis, I look forward to these activities and certainly love the competition. On the days I am not able to participate in these sports, I walk with my wife or other members of my family. Not only is this an excellent way to maintain fitness, but it is also wonderful for interpersonal relationships. When I have the opportunity to walk alone, I see this as an opportunity for education, so I use a set of headphones and listen to either a motivational tape or one of the many medical tapes to which I subscribe.

I know there is a dedicated band of people out there who detest all forms of exercise and, like our friend Oscar Wilde, would prefer to avoid the extra exertion at all costs. For those of you who fit this category, I would suggest a trade-off—do some form of routine, boring exercise while you're doing something you enjoy.

I will never forget an 88-year-old patient of mine who loved the daytime soapies on TV. I convinced her she needed an exercise program so she purchased a second-hand exercise bike and had it placed right in front of the television. She would start peddling at the start of *Days of Our Lives* and finish when *The Young and the Restless* began, performing this activity five days a week for an hour at a time (because the soapies are not on during the weekends). This wonderfully creative exercise program certainly contributed to her ongoing good health. Most of us can afford at least half an hour of television watching per day, so dust the old exercise bike off from the store room, and drag it into the lounge room. You may get complaints about the aesthetics, but no complaints about how you will feel in the long run with regular exercise.

DO YOU NEED TO JOG OR RUN TO BE TRULY FIT?

The answer to this is, of course, no. A good brisk walk is just as beneficial to your health as any other form of exercise and probably is less traumatic on your body.

IS THERE A REAL RISK FROM REGULAR RUNNING?

We occasionally hear of people who drop dead during their morning jog. The jog did not cause this, instead the trauma was due to some underlying condition that had not been detected. A study in the *Journal of the American College of Cardiology* that examined 50 000 runners participating in the Boston Marathon revealed a negligible rate of sudden cardiac death. Many more people die during sleep than during exercise. Does this mean we should not go to sleep at night?

If you are over the age of 35 and wish to start high-level exercise, I would suggest the following five strategies:

1. Have a thorough medical assessment, including a stress test (preferably a stress echo), with a full preventative screen to determine your cardiac risk.
2. Obtain sensible advice regarding correct footwear.
3. Avoid competing in a major race if you have had a flu-like illness during the two weeks before competition.
4. If you are suffering any new symptoms, such as fatigue, shortness of breath, dizziness or chest pain, consult your doctor immediately and don't compete in the race or do any exercise for the race.
5. If you are a regular long-distance runner, consult on a regular basis a sports physician, physio or trainer regarding sensible exercise to prevent or minimise injuries.

People with less personal motivation to exercise tend to find it easier to seek the help of a personal trainer, join a sporting team or enrol in a local gym. Some of the more creative services are providing an holistic approach with not only exercise facilities, but also massage and complementary health advice. Some of the larger medical practices also incorporate an holistic medicine service along with a gym and pre-exercise assessments. Whether it is using a personal trainer, attending a gym or joining a sporting team or facility that motivates you to exercise, it doesn't really matter—just as long as you keep exercising.

Quit smoking

During the early 1990s, I had the privilege of lecturing in six cities throughout mainland China. I was teaching cardiologists how to perform a new technique at that time known as transoesophageal echo. Transoesophageal echo is where a tube is inserted down the throat while the patient is under sedation, imaging the heart internally as the back of the heart is located in front of the oesophagus. These excellent pictures of the heart allow more accurate diagnoses of specific cardiac conditions.

I was in a hospital in Jinan, which is an eight-hour drive south-east of Beijing. After the lecture, I demonstrated a transoesophageal echo on a man in his forties who had severe rheumatic heart disease. One of the heart chambers, the left atrium, was almost completely full of clot. During this procedure there were about 20 cardiologists standing next to me around the examination couch and almost all of them were smoking.

I asked my interpreter to ask the doctors not to smoke, saying that in my country smoking in front of someone else is sometimes considered quite rude. The message I had back from the Chinese cardiologists was that in their country, if you don't smoke you're not a man. Unfortunately, this is the ethos in some countries. For those of us older than

40, we will recall that this was certainly the ethos in Western countries probably 20 to 30 years ago.

Clever advertising campaigns, such as those featuring 'the Malboro man', depicted rugged individuals who were 'tough' because they were smokers. I must state that there is nothing tough about wasting away to skin and bones and dying in pain—the actor in the Marlboro ad died of lung cancer. The famous Walt Disney died at the age of 66 of lung cancer, having been a heavy smoker for most of his life. What a pity that such a creative genius's life was cut short by a preventable disease. Fortunately, our attitudes to cigarette smoking have changed markedly since the Second World War.

During the war, many governments gave out free cigarettes as rations for soldiers, to provide comfort during the stressful times of war. Many doctors in the '40s and '50s used to suggest to people that they take up smoking as a form of stress relief. During this period it was almost normal for people to start smoking in their teens, and certainly the health effects of smoking were not at all well known or described.

Today, many parts of the United States, Canada and Australia have banned smoking in restaurants and public buildings. In fact, in many parts of these countries, you are made to feel a social outcast if you are a smoker. Unfortunately, however, there are still alarming rates of cigarette smoking among young people, especially young women. Young women, who are often so obsessed with their appearance, believe that cigarette smoke keeps them thin and also makes them more socially acceptable. But the rates of cigarette smoking in Europe and Asia (especially in India) are alarmingly high. It is interesting to note that the rates of cardiovascular disease and cancer are also increasing in these countries.

I must admit, however, there is nothing more irritating for the entrenched smoker to hear a reformed smoker talking about how they are a much stronger and better person because they could give the cigarettes away without any problems whatsoever. Around 50 years ago, probably 50 per cent of the adult population smoked. When many of these people heard of the increasing dangers of cigarette smoking, the ones who were not particularly addicted found it easy to kick the habit. Around one in five people in the community carry the gene for nicotine addiction. If you are one of the unlucky ones born with this gene and then become exposed to nicotine, it is very easy for you to become addicted.

The reasons people begin smoking in the first place are many, but the reasons people continue to smoke over the years are almost always related to nicotine addiction. I have seen far too many people who, despite significant cigarette-related illnesses, still could not stop smoking.

There is no logic to addiction. As part of my specialty training I worked for six months as a respiratory registrar. During this time, one of the professors of respiratory medicine, who advised people all day, every day that they should stop smoking, used to duck out at lunchtime for a cigarette—and he had already had coronary artery bypass grafting. Despite all the intellectual arguments in the world, if you are heavily addicted to nicotine, it is very difficult to kick the habit. We have all heard the stories of the person who lost both his legs from cigarette smoking, had his abdominal aortic aneurysm repaired (again related to cigarette smoking), had coronary artery bypass surgery and both his carotid arteries reamed out, but still smoked through his tracheostomy following the removal of his larynx for a cigarette smoking–related cancer. The only real solution would be to remove both hands so he could not light the cigarette in the first place!

I am always somewhat amused when I hear a smoker saying, 'I love my cigarettes. They relax me.' Well, what is the answer? Do cigarettes really relax somebody? The surprising answer to this is 'no'. Cigarettes are in fact, a stimulant. Nicotine is a significant stimulant but any smoker will tell you that they feel better and more relaxed when they have had their cigarette fix. There are a few physiological and psychological reasons for this.

The first physiological reason is that the centre of the brain that controls addiction is rather close to the centre of the brain that is stimulated during stress. When you feel stressed your addictive centre starts firing off and the first thing you want is to have your addiction calmed. Satisfying the addiction with nicotine will immediately calm this centre. The problem with having a nicotine fix, unfortunately, is that the half-life of nicotine is around 20 minutes to half an hour, so within half an hour or so you need another fix. This is why significantly addicted people can smoke anywhere between 20 to 40 cigarettes per day and often wake in the middle of the night needing and wanting another cigarette.

One of the other problems with cigarette smoking is that there is a direct link between nicotine addiction and depression. This is one of the explanations for why people who are depressed are often also smokers. This is also an explanation for why when someone stops smoking, they can often suffer a mild to moderate depressive illness. Of course, there are the psychological factors of the loss of the comfort of smoking, but there are, indeed, physiological changes when an interplay takes place between nicotine and serotonin levels. Serotonin is one of the major chemicals that is defective in people with depression. This is the basis for the action of the drug zyban.

Zyban was initially developed as an anti-depressant. When trialled for depression, many smokers would come into the researchers and say, 'You know, it's interesting . . . not only do I feel less depressed, but I've also lost the desire to smoke.' These clever researchers then started trialling zyban as a smoking cessation agent and, you guessed it, it worked very effectively. When zyban first came on the market there was a rush by many smokers to use this agent. This started to get the cigarette companies extremely worried and so, much misinformation was spread regarding the dangers of zyban. There were a few deaths, but what was not realised in these situations was that many smokers have underlying heart disease and many more smokers die from an acute heart attack while they are smoking than after they have withdrawn from cigarette smoking. If you write prescriptions for thousands and thousands of courses of zyban, there will always be a handful of people who will die while coincidentally taking the agent. The reason for this is that they have been long-term smokers and long-term smokers have higher death rates than non-smokers.

The only real caution with using zyban is if you have a past history of epilepsy. Zyban will significantly increase your risk of a fit in these circumstances. If you have not had epilepsy, it is extremely rare for a drug like zyban to cause this sort of problem.

Is zyban a cure? The answer to this is a definite 'no'. There is no drug for any condition that is a cure-all in every situation, just as there is no pharmaceutical agent that has no side effects. Whenever you take any treatment for any condition, there is always a risk. The sound doctor explains this risk but in discussing the condition or treatment with the patient, the most logical approach is to discuss the risks and benefits of the treatment versus the risks and benefits of not using the treatment. In the case of zyban, this is very clear. The benefits of using zyban are incredibly high. The risk of smoking cigarettes is extraordinarily high. In fact, in my long career of practising medicine, I have not seen any person towards the end of their smoking career who has said to me, 'You know, Doc, I'm really happy I took up smoking.' Universally, every patient laments the fact that they have been a cigarette smoker and wished they had either not gone anywhere near cigarettes or gave them up promptly in the beginning.

Cigarette smoking and metabolism

One of the great fears of most smokers, when they stop smoking, is weight gain. Why do people put on weight when they stop smoking? There are three possible explanations for this.

First, when you stop smoking, food definitely tastes better and your appetite returns. Therefore, without some degree of self-control you are quite likely to eat more food. Secondly, one of the psychological cues associated with cigarette smoking is the desire to have something in your mouth. If you don't have a cigarette in your mouth, which for years has given you a degree of psychological comfort, you may often replace this with putting food in your mouth. Even chewing on something can offer some psychological benefit. Unfortunately, if you put too much highly processed and packaged foods in your mouth you will put on weight; especially if you have just stopped smoking. Thirdly, metabolism. There is no doubt that cigarette smoking is a state of chronic poisoning. When you poison your system with cigarettes, you are basically driving up your basal metabolic rate. The cells, therefore, work faster and harder; but certainly not more efficiently. When you stop smoking there is a rebound slowing beyond normal of your metabolism. It is during the first three to six months after cessation of smoking that you are most likely to gain weight because of this marked slowing in your metabolism.

Think of it like this: chronic cigarette smoking is like a chronic illness, just like any chronic poisoning. If you swallowed a moderate, non-lethal dose of arsenic every day, over the months you would lose weight and become very ill. The poisons in cigarettes are like a slower form of arsenic. Instead of acute or sub-acute suicide, this is chronic suicide. It is, therefore, quite logical that when you stop this chronic insult to your body, your metabolism will rebound and initially slow. After six months, however, the metabolism is back to normal.

What, therefore, is the solution? The answer is to be careful when you stop smoking. If you do not follow the principles of Cell Factor nutrition—and I must say, stopping smoking is certainly one of those principles—your body will pay for it in some way or another. The most likely price to pay in this situation is weight gain. It is very important that you follow the nutritional principles and the exercise principles suggested in this book around the time you quit smoking.

There are two aspects to the desire to smoke. The first is the purely physical addictive aspect; and the second is the psychological habitual aspect. I remember a dear lady in her seventies who was one of my patients. She had severe emphysema and, no matter what she did, could not kick the smoking habit. One of the things doctors do not often do is ask people the circumstances of their smoking. I asked this lady exactly when and how she smoked. She said, 'I have a special chair in my house where I smoke.' On further questioning she went on to tell me that the chair was positioned so she had a lovely view of the river and she would walk in her door to her little safe haven, sit in her favourite chair looking over this view, and light a cigarette. You can see what I'm driving at—the psychological cues and comforts associated with the ritual of smoking in this fashion makes it very difficult to break the habit.

Another one of my patients, this one in her sixties, had associated high blood pressure and some early heart problems related to smoking. She told me, 'Doctor, I *love* my cigarettes.' Even the use of the word 'love' in association with cigarettes means there is a strong psychological bond to the habit of smoking. When I asked further about how she smoked, she was quick to tell me that her family was so disgusted with her habit, that she was not allowed to smoke anywhere near the house. She was banished to the back garden. She was very happy to add that she loved being sent out, away from the rabble inside the house to the solitude of the back garden. She would take the newspaper, a cup of coffee and a cigarette and sit in the garden enjoying every moment. Again, without breaking these psychological cues, it is very, very difficult to convince someone to stop smoking.

The facts about smoking

As much as I'd love to give smokers an 'out', I'm afraid all the bad press about cigarette smoking is absolutely justified. There are well over 40 major poisons in one cigarette. Every time you smoke a cigarette you are taking these poisons to every cell in your body. The smoking of one cigarette generates *3 trillion* free radicals in your bloodstream. If you combine this with living in a polluted city (and let's face it, most of us do these days), the statistics are even worse. There are also many people who work in rather difficult environmental circumstances. Working in mines, being exposed to asbestos, working on dusty building sites and working with chemicals or other forms of wood-based dusts and grains can exacerbate the effects of cigarette smoking.

Every year in the United States, there are around 2 million deaths. Of this figure, 400 000 are directly attributable to cigarette smoke. An even more alarming statistic is that 57 000 of these 400 000 deaths are due to passive cigarette smoking. Another alarming statistic is that because smokers can no longer smoke at their desk, they are ducking out for a cigarette every hour or two. The lost productivity from the absent smoker amounts to around $5000 per smoker per year.

Probably the least poisonous of the poisons in cigarettes, but certainly the main addictive part, is nicotine. Nicotine is a stimulant and highly addictive, but by itself probably does not cause much in the way of disease. It is certainly used as replacement therapy for smoking—with great success. Most people who attempt nicotine patches or gum find them of benefit. One of my good friends, who has quite significant asthma and stopped smoking 14 years ago, has remained severely addicted to nicotine gum. He chews quite a few pieces every day but has not returned to cigarettes. Whether this is causing him long-term health problems or not is yet to be seen but, certainly, the use of the patch or the gums or the inhalant is a better alternative to smoking itself.

In my opinion, and in the opinion of many other experts, the best form of nicotine replacement is the patch. This gives a small, graded dose of nicotine throughout the day, which allows the smoker to have their nicotine addiction satisfied, but eventually it makes it easier to come off nicotine completely. If you chew gum, a large dose of nicotine is delivered to your bloodstream, somewhat similar to that of smoking. This makes it more difficult to stop using the gum. In fact, the best way to use gum, if you wish to have this as your cessation method, is to keep the gum in your mouth and occasionally bite on it to allow smaller doses of nicotine to travel into your system. Probably the least effective form of nicotine replacement is the inhalant. This absolutely simulates cigarette smoking and makes it very difficult to stop the inhalant completely.

One of the great con-jobs of the tobacco industry is low-tar versus high-tar and low-nicotine versus high-nicotine cigarettes. With a supposedly 'lite' cigarette, highly addicted smokers will simply inhale more deeply to get a better 'hit' from the cigarette. They will also smoke more of the cigarette to take in more nicotine. All this does is deliver more combustible substances, such as carbon monoxide and benzpyrene, to the outer parts of the lungs, causing more damage and predisposing the smoker to cancer. The only safe cigarette is no cigarette at all.

Benzpyrene and other parts of the tar are the probable cancer-producing parts of the cigarette. Although lung cancer is the most commonly associated cancer, there are many other types of cancers—such as cancers of the mouth, tongue and other areas of the gastro-intestinal tract, and cancer of the bladder—that are also strongly associated with cigarette smoking. If you wrap your lips around an exhaust pipe and suck in the fumes, one of the main emissions, carbon monoxide, will cause you all sorts of enormous problems. You probably would take in about the same amount of carbon monoxide in a cigarette as you would from an exhaust pipe.

Carbon monoxide by itself is a deadly poison causing severe problems with the oxygen-carrying component of your bloodstream (haemoglobin). It also causes a marked vaso constriction. Constriction of blood vessels is a potentially life-threatening problem. There is a condition known as coronary artery spasm, where a supposedly normal artery goes into spasm and can even shut down completely, causing a heart attack. Eighty per cent of people who suffer coronary artery spasm are long-term smokers. The combination of carbon monoxide and the enormous amount of free radicals generated by a cigarette is a major factor in the generation of coronary heart disease.

Case study: Bert—One of the most upsetting moments in my medical career came when Bert, a 42-year-old, 40-cigarette-a-day smoker was admitted under my care to a coronary unit. The main artery in his heart was blocked, causing one of the largest heart attacks I have ever seen anyone survive, but he was not surviving particularly well. His systolic blood pressure was running at about 60 mmHg, which is extremely low. He was hardly getting any blood into his tissues. We had the transplant team mobilised but it was impossible to wheel him out of the room, let alone get him to surgery for a heart transplant if a donor heart became available, because every time we tried to move him in any way, shape or form, he would develop a serious heart rhythm known as ventricular tachycardia. His heart would stop beating and, over the three-day period he survived, he required about 60 electric shocks to get his heart back to normal.

After the third day, our efforts failed and he died. I was given the job to explain to his wife that her six small children no longer had a father. I listened to this bereaved family in disbelief plead and beg with me to do something. But, of course, I couldn't bring him back to life. I must admit, I went home after this tragedy and cried myself because I felt so helpless.

This man died of a totally preventable disease. Cigarette smoke–induced disease is not an old person's disease. Cigarette smokers die on average 10 to 15 years younger than non-smokers. They have a four times higher rate of heart disease, an eight times higher rate of sudden death and a 300 times higher rate of lung cancer.

Joan Simmons was 36 years old. When she was a child, both of her parents smoked. When she left home at 18, she herself took up smoking. At the age of 36 she coughed up blood and a chest X-ray revealed a mass on the left lung. After further testing it was decided to remove her left lung and she had the typical squamous cell cancer of the lung, one of the two common cigarette-associated lung cancers.

You will hear smokers say, 'Yeah, but non-smokers also get lung cancer. My grandmother never smoked at all and she developed lung cancer.' The answer to this is that Grandpa was probably a smoker and she developed the lung cancer as a consequence of Grandpa's smoking.

In the case of Joan, she was now in her mid-thirties with one lung that was also damaged by cigarettes. She was given a course of radiotherapy and around two years later suffered a heart attack. The heart attack was probably a consequence of the combination of cigarette smoking and some radiation-induced coronary disease (this is a well-described phenomenon). The heart attack was quite extensive, involving the front wall of the heart. Joan now had a heart that was working at around 50 per cent of its capability and one lung that was also working at around 50 per cent of its capacity. This young woman had severe heart and lung disease *strongly* related to her parents' smoking habit and her subsequent smoking habit. A situation that was totally preventable.

Smokers looking for justification for their habit will say, 'My uncle is now 80 years old and has smoked all of his life and has never had any problems.' Of course, there will always be exceptions to the rule. I have also seen people in their eighties who have smoked without any obvious problems. When I assessed them, though, I didn't think they were par-ticularly healthy—they were usually struggling at the age of 80 to breathe and be mobile. But, yes, this does occasionally happen. The figures are very straightforward: around 60 per cent of smokers will develop some form of chronic lung disease. This can be either in the form of chronic bronchitis, which is basically coughing sputum for at least three to six months of the year, or as emphysema. Emphysema is basically the process whereby cigarettes destroy the air sacks, causing shortness of breath with minimal activity.

If you have a history of asthma, bronchitis or one of the related disorders as a child, you have a 100 per cent chance of developing some form of chronic lung disease as you age. If you smoke through your lifetime you have a 60 per cent chance of developing coronary heart disease and around a 20 per cent chance of developing lung cancer. It takes one lung cancer cell nine years to become 2 centimetres wide, then six months to become a 2-kilogram-size tumour. This is the tumour-doubling rate.

If you make the decision to stop smoking today, within three months your risk of sudden cardiac death has stopped, and within two years your risk of coronary heart disease has been markedly reduced, almost back to that of a non-smoker. It is very unlikely that you will develop lung cancer if after 10 years of not smoking you have not had a problem. You will probably also regain somewhere between 5 and 10 per cent of your lung function, no matter when you stopped smoking.

What I am saying is very straightforward. There is *always* a benefit to stopping smoking, regardless of your age. Obviously, the earlier you stop, the better off you are, but even in your sixties, seventies or eighties you will derive some relief and benefit from not smoking.

How to quit

So, I've scared the life out of you and you've made the decision that you want to stop smoking. How do you go about it? I believe there are five aspects of quitting smoking:

1. desire
2. support
3. pharmacological help
4. tailored messages (health tailoring)
5. five-point action plan.

1. DESIRE

If you have *absolutely* no desire to stop smoking, I can promise you—you won't stop smoking. Even if there is a slight seed in your head that is gnawing away at you saying, 'You know, I really shouldn't be doing this . . .' then at least that's a start. Often the desire to stop smoking is precipitated by some acute life event. A common life event can be one of the following:

- Meeting a new partner who can't stand smoking.
- Finding out you're pregnant.
- Developing acute illness, such as a heart attack or severe pneumonia.
- Your best friend, who is a smoker, suddenly drops dead.
- You lose your job and you can no longer afford to buy cigarettes.

I could go on with a multitude of reasons and, frankly, I don't care what the reason is—as long as something will prompt you to want to stop smoking.

2. SUPPORT

If you deside you want to stop smoking, it is important that you make a public declaration to those around you that you are going to stop smoking—even if you are surrounded by smokers. If they are smokers, it is important you ask them to be supportive and respectful of your decision. If they are not smokers, ask them to be patient and not to expect too much. It may take you quite a few attempts to stop. The most important thing is that you are trying and that you will continue to try until you have succeeded.

PROFESSIONAL COACH

Part of your support system could be to have a detached, professional person who can guide you through smoking cessation. One of Australia's top smoking cessation experts is Dr Renee Bittoun in Sydney. Renee's success at helping people quit smoking is much higher than many other health professionals, and to engage the help of an expert such as Renee can make quitting so much easier.

One of the important aspects of taking on a professional coach to help you stop smoking is the aspect of follow-up. It is human nature that, for the first few days to weeks, we will be highly motivated; but then when some usual life stress crops up or we perform some high-risk behaviour, we often slip back into old habits. This is, of course, very typical if you have rather unsupportive, cigarette-smoking friends who do not like you stepping outside their 'club'.

It is human nature to want people to think and feel as we do. This is no different for smokers. If your smoking friends see that you want to stop smoking and they're not ready to make that sort of commitment to themselves, they will often make you feel as if you are letting *them* down by pursuing this course. Often in this situation, a smoking friend will feel a personal slight, believing that you feel you are better than them because you are stopping smoking.

This is where the professional coach is important. Follow-up is something that is sadly lacking from many professional services. We all have that warm-fuzzy feeling from the initial service, but this soon disappears when we merge back into our normal life patterns.

3. PHARMACOLOGICAL HELP

The professional coach is usually in the best position to give you the correct advice as to what type of pharmacological support, in terms of patches, gum, inhalant or drugs, you will need to stop smoking. Although there is no restriction to your using the patches without any help, it is much better to have professional advice and professional supervision when using any pharmacological substance. It is my opinion that it is very difficult to stop smoking without some pharmacological support, and I certainly would not see this as a slight on you as a smoker, and it does not imply you are weaker than other smokers who give up without the use of pharmacology. To think this way is almost like a person who has high blood pressure saying, 'I can beat blood pressure without pills.' This is a ridiculous argument as blood pressure is a metabolic problem that needs metabolic adjustments with medications in almost all cases.

4. HEALTH TAILORING

The concept of health tailoring is very simple. The retail industry came to understand tailoring many, many years ago. There is certainly no one-size-fits-all when it comes to wearing clothes, nor is there when tailoring a health program. Health tailoring is particularly useful for smoking cessation. One of the world experts in health tailoring is a colleague of mine, Dr Vic Strecher, from Ann Arbor, Michigan, in the United States. I visited Dr Strecher's laboratory a few years back and was extremely impressed by his innovative techniques.

Strecher's team has developed a computerised system known as the 'health kiosk'. This is basically a touch-pad computer screen that is now being placed in large shopping centres or on-site in large corporations around America. Using the simple touch-pad screen, the person involved answers a series of questions with a series of options. This option allows you to determine where you are in your smoking phase; what are your roadblocks or the behavioural situations that are preventing you from stopping smoking, the particular situations and reasons why you are smoking; and the tailored ways in which you can help kick the habit. A combination of desire, support, pharmacology, and a tailored message markedly increases the chance of success of a quit-smoking program, and not just in the short term.

Ten to 15 years ago, many institutions offered five-day quit-smoking plans. These were highly successful over the first week with a 90 per cent quit rate, but when these people were reviewed 12 months later, only 5 per cent were still non-smokers. The newer programs have up to a 60 to 70 per cent 12-month success rate. Unfortunately, there will always be the ingrained smoker who, no matter *what* is offered, will continue to smoke. Nobody's perfect!

5. FIVE-POINT ACTION PLAN

The five-point action plan involves:

(i) decision
(ii) interrupt the limiting patterns
(iii) create a new pattern

(iv) condition the pattern

(v) live the program.

Decision: Without a decision to change, nothing will change. If we don't make this decision and make the decision very public, and even to the point of writing down this decision in a journal, then I believe any attempt to quit smoking is doomed for failure.

Interrupt the limiting patterns: Unfortunately, we're confronted with many situations that will make stopping smoking very difficult. For example, if it is your habit to visit the pub on a Friday night and drink with your friends, after a few glasses of alcohol your ability to say 'no' to a cigarette will be reduced. For the first few weeks after making the decision to stop, you may need to stop your Friday pub nights until you have ingrained your new pattern. You might have a particular chair or place where you smoke which is associated with relaxation and pleasure. This needs to change. Often, I say to my patients, 'Yes, you can smoke if you want, but you must smoke in front of your house while people are walking past. Face the wall and look rather silly.' Often the embarrassment of doing this is enough to make people want to stop.

It may even come down to taking the drastic step of ending a relationship before you are prepared to give up smoking. Often, someone may be involved in a toxic relationship, and smoking is part of that toxicity. Only you know what is stopping you from quitting smoking, and you know how you can change and interrupt that limiting pattern.

Case study: Nick—A 33-year-old man named Nick came to see me for a heart check-up. Nick was a 20-cigarette-a-day man but he was actually quite disgusted with his smoking habit and keen on stopping. He did, however, say to me, 'I *love* smoking.' I found out that Nick's father had died at the age of 42, when Nick was 14, of sudden cardiac death related to smoking. I asked Nick about the funeral, how he felt while he was sitting in the church. He answered, 'It was the worst moment of my life.'

Nick had two small children aged nine and six. He was a

devoted father. I then hit Nick below the belt with what I believed to be a fairly confronting technique. I said to him that if he was really serious about giving up cigarettes, whenever he felt like smoking he should visualise a church and a coffin. In the coffin would be Nick's dead body. Sitting in the front row would be his two children, crying—feeling the same pain Nick felt when his father died. I then said, 'Nick, if you *truly* love your children and you don't want them to suffer that pain, you *must* stop smoking and use this visualisation technique to help.' He used the technique and was able to stop smoking.

Create a new pattern: This is the pleasure/pain principle. You must associate enormous pain with your current habit—as in the case of Nick in the above case study—but also associate enormous pleasure with not smoking. The best and easiest way to do this is to create a bank account and discipline yourself to save the money you would've otherwise spent on cigarettes. Instead of this money 'going up in smoke', it is building up in a bank account. At the end of 12 months you can then withdraw the money and spend it on something you want, such as a holiday or a deposit on a new car, or even a whole new wardrobe. It doesn't matter what you do, but it is important that you associate pleasure with your new pattern. You must reward yourself in some way in order to reinforce not smoking.

Condition the new pattern: Not only do you need to see your bank account grow when you stop smoking, but you also have to realise that, especially for the first month, it is important you have strong willpower. One of the greatest principles of self-discipline is delayed gratification. When you really feel like smoking, put off the desire and become busy with something else. After a while, you may find the desire weakens because you've been able to exhibit delayed gratification. After a month of conditioning the new pattern, it will be a lot easier.

Live the program: You have made the decision to become a non-smoker. You have disciplined yourself by interrupting limiting patterns and creating the new pattern and doing that one month of hard work to create a new habit that does not involve smoking. It is now important that you realise this is a lifelong program. Bad things will happen in your life—as they do with all of us—and it is important you weather these storms. Realise that the cessation of smoking cigarettes is one of the most profound and health-promoting actions you can ever take.

The Cell Factor program does not just involve eating the right foods or exercise. It involves treating all of your cells with the utmost respect. No mater how healthy your food, no matter how many supplements you swallow every day, and no matter how much exercise you do—if you are bombarding your cells with toxic cigarette smoke you cannot achieve Cell Factor nutrition. I have never, and will never, see a healthy cigarette smoker. But I have seen many healthy non-smokers and maybe, in your case, ex-smokers.

Manage your stress

Is stress a condition that can cripple you physically, mentally, emotionally and spiritually? Or is it just the yuppie disease of our age?

Stress is defined in the dictionary as a 'great pressure or strain'. In his book *Man's Search for Meaning*, Viktor Frankl argues that life's stressful events actually give us a reason to exist. Professor Frankl was tortured in a Nazi concentration camp for about two years. When he was released from the camp he bore no bitterness and didn't plunge into alcoholism or drug addiction, but set off with a new challenge in life. From his experiences in the camp he formulated what has become known as logo therapy, or 'living through meaning': it is not the stress, but the way you handle it, that is important.

Ten thousand years ago, humans lived in a rather wild and dangerous world. Because of the dangers of the time, ancient man needed his wits about him. Our body had developed two automatic systems to cope with the extremes of danger and the extremes of relaxation, such as a deep sleep.

The fear–fight–flight system, otherwise known as the sympathetic nervous system, would switch into action with a pending attack from a sabre-tooth tiger or a neighbouring tribe. This fear–fight–flight system made the heart beat faster and harder, delivering more blood flow to the muscles and widening the pupils. This allowed the person to have a greater field of vision and greater strength in his muscles to either defend himself or run. Without this system, it might take a few minutes for the heart to generate enough force to deliver increased blood flow to the muscles. By this time our ancient friend would be the main course at some primitive feline banquet.

Conversely, the last thing any of us need when we are in a deep sleep is a torrential blood flow through our muscles or a heart that is jumping out of our chest. The opposite, or parasympathetic nervous system, winds the system down. The pulse slows, the blood pressure drops and the blood flow to the non-functioning muscles becomes a trickle, like a river after a three-year drought. This conserves energy, which is also an important part of survival.

Of course, our modern-day stress factors are different (to some extent), but our physical responses to them are the same. However, if you live in a society such as ours, there are many external pressures or strains that cause varying degrees of *reactions* from different people. Some will feel extremely anxious, both inwardly and outwardly; to an external observer, they will be accused of being stressed. Another person may not seem overtly stressed by a particular situation, but internally will be suffering great angst. This can manifest as a whole host of physical or psychological symptoms.

REASONS FOR STRESS

I believe there are five major reasons stress is increasing in a society where all of the technological benefits should be making our life easier:

1. choice
2. instant answers
3. multiskilling
4. work security
5. litigation.

1. Choice

Strange as it may seem, having excessive choices are a great cause of stress. You can no longer walk into a cafe to order a cup of coffee without making somewhere between four and 10 choices. Do you want a cappuccino, a flat white, a short black, a long black, or just standard filtered coffee? Do you want full-cream milk, skim milk, soy milk? Normal sugar, raw sugar or artificial sweetener? What size do you want—small, medium or large? Do you want to drink the coffee in the cafe or take it away. The final insult comes when you are asked, 'How do you want to pay for that? Cash, credit card or eftpos?' And that's for just a cup of coffee!

2. Instant answers

With today's global marketplace and global communication, there is an incredible need for instant answers. Most people in the corporate world work bizarre hours so that they keep in touch with the markets around the world. It is not unusual for late-night video conferencing or tele-conferences, and it is certainly taken for granted that instant answers/solutions are expected. This takes away the ability for careful contemplation and many bad decisions are made because of hastily cobbled-together solutions, purely to satisfy this thirst for instant answers. The need to think this quickly puts enormous pressure on everyone, but with the 'Emperor's New Clothes' scenario that has encompassed the modern corporate world, no-one seems to be standing up and saying, 'Hey fellas, this is *ridiculous.*'

3. Multiskilling

Although many areas of the world are becoming increasingly specialised, often these specialists are expected to be multiskilled as well. In my field of medicine, 40 to 50 years ago we only had the pink pills and the green ones—which were usually both the same. These days, just for a condition such as high blood pressure, there are over 50 different drugs from which to choose. The actions and side effects and dose ranges of all of these pills need to be well known before prescribing, so we now have specialists in high blood pressure. Within my field of cardiology there are specialties within specialties. My specialty happens to be preventative cardiology and heart scanning. There are interventional cardiologists who spend most of their time putting stents and balloons in blocked arteries.

Despite this, many specialists working in large hospitals also have to spend many hours in administration, dealing with emails and typing.

4. Work security

Most of us like our creature comforts, and part of our creature comforts is security. We find security in matters familiar. Change creates many situations with which we are not familiar and, thus, increases our stress levels. On a work level, the concepts of profits before people and concern for the happiness of the shareholder rather than the happiness of the worker have become the norm, the new paradigm. This creates an enormous sense of unease and dissatisfaction for not only workers, but executives and CEOs.

I believe over the next few years we will continue to see many corporations crumble as the short-term gain of restructuring and shaving off human carcasses for pure profit continues. You only have to look to Japan to see how the corporate dedication and ethic has culled so many people, causing insecurity among the population that many Japanese workers will no longer tolerate the attitude of 'live to work', they now 'work to live'. This persistent change in our lives is in many ways destroying the balance, and it is my opinion that human beings can only tolerate so much.

5. Litigation

The threat of being sued for a major or minor misdemeanour is often in the back of a worker's mind. In my field in medicine there are not too many people that haven't been involved in litigation, whether for unfair or justified reasons. Many of my colleagues have suffered enormous stress for what I believe to be completely unjustified actions on the part of the plaintiff. Often, these legal challenges are because people refuse to take responsibility for their own actions, but, suffice to say, this still causes enormous stress for everyone involved.

I well remember a patient who was challenging the Veterans' Administration Board in Australia (known as the Department of Veterans' Affairs). This particular gentleman spent three years of his life floating all manner of legal challenges against the department for what I personally felt was not a particularly justifiable claim. The legal fight itself had dragged him down personally and for the minimal amount of gain he received after the years of anguish, stress and personality change this caused, it was certainly not worth it.

PATHOLOGICAL EFFECTS

All these five factors have created an artificial situation in our society, placing more stress on people than ever before. But interestingly, many people crumble under this stress while others thrive in it. I do have the belief that being exposed to these excessive amounts of stress levels will exact some sort of price. When you look at the spectrum of psychological disorders in our society, from neuroses to road rage, we can see that price.

Our reaction to stress is never straightforward and usually it depends on many factors, including our early childhood training, our inherent personality and the true impact of the particular stress on our lives when it occurs at the time. One of the big issues, however, is not just *how* stress affects us psychologically, but how it can also contribute or even *cause* many of the common diseases with which we are afflicted. As with most aspects of medicine, there is no good answer to this question. World experts on the subject have fought tooth and nail, jealously guarding their position based on their own prejudices and experiences.

During the attack on the World Trade Center on 11 September 2001 and the earthquakes in Los Angeles in 1994, the rates of heart attack, stroke and sudden death increased seven times the average rate. Most people would agree that stress can certainly precipitate an event in someone who is destined to suffer that event. On the other hand, the death rate during Chinese New Year is much lower than the period soon after, indicating that looking forward to a special date can help ward off death by possibly the reverse mechanism.

None of these events really answer the question as to whether there is a causative aspect to stress or purely a precipitative aspect. When you seek to understand what truly causes something, it is usually not due to a single explanation. It is very unusual in life for one particular cause to be the absolute explanation. You could argue that a person's genes cause a condition, but there are often other factors, such as stressors that go with that. The children of a person afflicted with Huntington's chorea have a 50 per cent chance of developing the disease. This is one of the only situations in life where if you have the gene you will definitely get the condition. Most other diseases, however, have a multi-factorial causation, with genetics being just one of the factors.

I have no doubt that stress is a major contributor to disease. Often, people who suffer heart attacks are under enormous stress and, interestingly, the most common time for a heart attack is eight o'clock, Monday morning. Think about it. Obviously, it was not the bus trip into work that caused the heart attack, there are many other factors that are operative in someone's life. I am sure the acute stress of going to work after a pleasant weekend is one of the factors.

There is now increasing scientific evidence that psycho-social factors contribute to the development of heart disease. I would like to summarise a brilliant review by Professor Rozanski and his colleagues from one of the premier cardiac journals, *Circulation*, where he discussed the impact of psychological factors on the generation of heart disease. Basically, his group suggested that there are five specific areas that show a significant relation to the acceleration, aggravation and possible causation of coronary heart disease. These areas were:

1. depression
2. anxiety
3. character and personality traits
4. social isolation
5. chronic life stressors.

Professor Rozanski's group goes on to discuss the two possible mechanisms for this relationship. The first is that anyone on the wrong side of any of these five areas has a higher likelihood of adverse health behaviours, such as poor diet, cigarette smoking and lack of exercise, that would contribute to the generation of heart disease. Even more concerning, but equally as important, is the fact that any of these five factors can contribute to direct pathological effects, such as the stimulation of the nerves and hormones involved in stress, or an alteration in the factors in the bloodstream that lead to inflammation and clotting.

1. Depression

Depression is a very common problem in our society. It is estimated that at any one time, one in 20 people suffers a major depression. In patients with coronary artery disease, the rate of depression is, in fact, three times higher.

Depression is characterised by a depressed mood and a significant lack of interest in most activities. This persists for at least two weeks and is usually associated with some of the following symptoms:

- change in appetite
- sleep disturbance
- fatigue
- slowing of activity or agitation
- feelings of guilt or worthlessness
- concentration problems
- suicidal thoughts.

There have been numerous scientific studies showing a close relationship between depression as being a major factor in the causation of cardiac disease in otherwise healthy people and the precipitation of further cardiac events in people with existing heart disease. Even if people are not depressed, the presence of any of the associated depressive symptoms above is associated with a higher risk for cardiac events.

Of particular interest is the sympton of hopelessness—the feeling that life is worthless and there is no hope for the future—has been associated with sudden death. A phenomenon known as vital exhaustion is characterised by the triad of fatigue, irritability and demoralised feelings.

There has been a strong association between vital exhaustion and cardiac events in healthy and coronary heart disease populations.

There is no doubt that people tend to follow a poor diet, smoke more and do not exercise when they are depressed. There are also three other direct mechanisms that occur and are associated with depression. The first is an elevation in the stress hormone, cortisone. Cortisone elevated over a period of time can weaken blood vessels and rupture established plaques. The second mechanism is altered platelet function. Platelets are the sticky elements in the bloodstream that form clots with the protein clotting factors. Platelets become much more sticky during periods of depression and predisposed to clots forming, especially in the coronary arteries.

Finally, there is a syndrome known as heart-rate variability. This is the ability of our heart to respond normally to different circumstances, such as stress or relaxation. If this variability is impaired, our parasympathetic, or relaxation, system does not function properly and we have an increased risk for rhythm disturbance in our heart. This commonly occurs in depressed patients.

The reason for this rather long-winded explanation of depression is to demonstrate the link between a seemingly psychological syndrome and the ways the presence of this syndrome can affect Cell Factor nutrition. If our cells are flooded with cortisone, such as in the case of depression, or the blood supply to the cells is sluggish, as occurs in depression when the platelets are switched on, then our metabolism and nutrition is affected. As depression is such a common problem, and increasingly so in our society, it is vital it is recognised and treated early so we can maintain our path towards Cell Factor nutrition.

2. Anxiety

One of our character traits is that we like an explanation for everything. I don't know how many times I've seen patients in my practice who state categorically that whatever disease they have been struck down with it is related to a particular occurrence. I'll see someone with severe lung disease who will relate it to an episode of inhaling some alleged toxic poison. This for them will be the cause of their lung disease, completely ignoring their lifelong cigarette habit as a possible factor.

One of the greatest causes for most of life's ills is the day-to-day anxieties many of us suffer. There is a very strong tendency for people to blame their work environment for their anxieties and their subsequent health problems. Unfortunately, in our increasingly litigious world, people feel that they should have compensation for whatever condition they suffer. For example, the man with the strong family history of heart disease, cholesterol abnormalities and high blood pressure who has an argument with someone at work, collapses and has a heart attack may then wish to sue his employer, claiming it was the acute stress of the argument that brought on the attack. The issue here is how much should we blame acute precipitants for the cause of conditions. I do not believe there is any major dispute within the medical profession that it is acute anxieties that are the final straw in the generation of some disease process.

As I have mentioned, on the day of the attack on the World Trade Center in New York City, the rates of heart attack, stroke and sudden death was seven times higher. What I failed to mention was that for a few weeks after these attacks, the rates were lower. The reason for this is that the people who were going to die or suffer these conditions at some stage in the next few months were all precipitated by the acute, severe tragedy of September 11. Therefore, the people that were already waiting for their condition had the acute precipitant on that day. That does not mean that the September 11 attack *caused* the heart attack, but it was obviously the precipitant for a condition that was almost certainly going to occur anyhow.

The big unanswered question is not whether acute anxieties, or even chronic anxieties, can precipitate a problem, but, can they contribute to the cause of the problem through either aggravating, exacerbating or accelerating the underlying condition?

There have been three large-scale community-based studies involving around 34 000 men (unfortunately, done only with men). These have shown a direct link between anxiety disorders and cardiac death. Even more concerning is that these studies have shown the more the anxiety, the more the chance of cardiac death. Strangely enough, however, there is not an association between anxiety and heart attack in these studies.

In fact, most of the death rates were due to sudden death; *not* non-sudden cardiac death. (As I have stated before in this book, a cardiac arrest is not the same as a heart attack. When the heart stops beating, the persons drops to the ground suddenly and unless they are resuscitated or the heart spontaneously restarts, they will die.) What this is implying is that acute and, more commonly, chronic anxiety disorders, and the direct inference from this, chronic stress, can build up to the point where an acute arrhythmia (rhythm disturbance in the heart) can stop the heart beating, leading to a cardiac arrest.

Again, I see a problem with many of these psychological studies. It is very difficult to say how much stress is affecting one particular person. I see many people in my practice who freely admit to me they don't suffer stress but I find them enormously anxious about their health and about their life in general. I see other people who really do not appear to be under particular stress at all but freely admit that they are incredibly anxious and worried about their health—even if they really have nothing to worry about at all. The point I am making is that it is extremely difficult to make judgment about stress levels and how those stress levels are affecting any one particular person.

Doctors love numbers. A number such as a cholesterol level can be measured, followed and treated. And even though many people over the years have attempted to quantify anxiety, depression and a whole host of other psychological symptoms with different anxiety and depression scales, there is still a strong degree of subjectivity—some would argue personal dishonesty—in the answers given to the questions. There is the age-old saying that 'It is the squeaky wheel that gets the oil.' Therefore, 'It is the patient that complains of a symptom that gets attention.' It is also the person that complains of a symptom that is brought to the attention of the profession. I often wonder how many people out there are suffering in silence and never get treatment programs, but live with their anxiety or depression for many years having come to accept this as almost normal.

Although the mind–body connection has become much more accepted these days, psychological and psychiatric diseases are still the realm of the psychologist and the psychiatrist. I strongly believe, though, that a person's life situation, including their acute and chronic stressors, their own inherent personality and their degree of emotional support, does have a powerful influence—not only on their own personal contentment, but also on the type and severity of diseases for with they are afflicted. Unfortunately, there will probably never be a concensus in the medical field as to the degree of contribution.

3. Character and personality traits

In the '60s, two psychologists came out with personality classifications that were very broad. There was the 'type-A' and the 'type-B' person. The type-A person was the driven perfectionist who was usually rather successful work-wise. This person is more specifically characterised as being highly competitive, hostile and bearing an exaggerated commitment to work. The type-B person was seen more as the lazy slob who couldn't wait until the bell rang at 5 p.m. so he could visit the pub, have a few beers, then go home and watch television. The research from the two psychologists strongly suggests that the type-A person was much more prone to heart attack, stroke and other forms of cardiovascular disease. The type-B person, however, did not appear to suffer these diseases as much.

When these results were more carefully analysed, however, it appeared that it was a sub-group of type-A that was more prone to cardiovascular disease. This was the type-A person who also happened to be time-urgent, hostile and angry. This is the fool who beeps his horn in peak-hour traffic despite the fact that blowing your horn in this situation really doesn't get the traffic moving any faster. It is the person who comes into my clinic and within 30 seconds of arriving is complaining about the time he's had to wait because he's a busy man and he doesn't have the time to waste sitting in a doctor's surgery.

A study showed that within two hours of becoming acutely angry with anyone, your risk for a heart attack increases 100 times. There is a wonderful Buddhist saying: 'You are not punished *for* your anger, you are punished *by* your anger.' So being a hostile, angry person is really a major risk factor for heart disease. Not only does hostility lead to unhealthy lifestyle behaviour, but it also increases the heart rate and blood pressure. People who are hostile have been shown to have high levels of cortisol and other stress hormones, such as adrenaline.

4. Social isolation

Whether you study animals in the wild, in the zoo or in the human race, most enjoy social contact. Most of us like being accepted by our group and it is a common human trait to seek the approval of others. There have been quite a few studies that show how people who are part of a traditional ethnic group tend to have higher rates of coronary artery disease if they leave the group for some reason or have been ostracised by the group. A study of animals in the Philadelphia Zoo who were exposed to overcrowding and social disruption showed a tenfold increase in fat build-up in their arteries, compared with animals in their natural environment.

5. Chronic life stressors

The work environment is a common source of stress for many people. 'Job strain', which is a situation of high work demand but low job control, has been shown in different studies to contribute significantly to the risk of cardiac disease. Of course, we all need money and in many situations it is difficult for a worker to change jobs. I must state, however, that I do not believe any one life situation will bring on a heart attack. You must bear some degree of personal responsibility and decision-making regarding your future, rather than blame your employer.

Probably one of the greatest life stresses is the death of a loved one. The death of a lifelong partner, the death of a parent or, even worse, the death of a child can have profound effects both on the psyche and on the health of the individual.

Vera is one of my 74-year-old patients whose husband died five years ago. Since his death, she has endured coronary artery bypass grafting, severe high blood pressure and recurrent rhythm disturbances in her heart. She has also had bladder problems and constantly feels tired. Before the death of her husband she was perfectly well and hardly ever attended doctors.

When someone close to you dies, or a long-term relationship splits up, it is easy for people who are not directly involved to say, 'Time will heal all wounds'; but for many people, it is very difficult to recover from a situation such as this.

So many people are trapped in situations somewhat beyond their control. There are many marriages where one partner has the financial control and tends to wield this control over the other partner. The other partner is trapped often because of children and lack of funds, and has to make the decision to either leave and attempt to become financially independent, which in some cases causes more hardship than the alternative.

One of the most important healing processes is to allow the grief reaction to occur. Many people feel they should suppress their acute response and 'be strong'. It is very important to confront the stress and allow whatever acute emotional reaction you are having to occur. Find a sympathetic relative or friend who will cry with you, get angry (if it is justified), and allow time to heal some of the wounds.

There are numerous studies, most of which show a significant relationship between poor social support, social isolation and other factors, such as chronic emotional trauma, that have been associated with the risk of significant medical illnesses such as cardiovascular disease and cancer. I have no doubt that in many cases it is our reaction to our situation rather than the situation itself that determines not only our psychological outcome, but also our health outcome after an acute or chronic life trauma.

STRESS MANAGEMENT

For many of us dealing with our normal day-to-day traumas, the so-called expected peaks and troughs of life, it is important that we have mechanisms that allow our life to function as smoothly as it possibly can. My five-point plan for a stress-free life is:

1. goal-setting
2. coping mechanisms
3. relationships
4. creative techniques
5. action.

1. Goal-setting

We need to set goals in the five aspects of our life. These aspects are physical, mental, emotional, financial and spiritual. In a study of Harvard graduates followed for 10 years, those who wrote down specific and clear goals in each of these areas were much more successful than those who didn't. Only 3 per cent of the graduates wrote clear, specific goals. At the end of 10 years they had earned more money than the other 97 per cent put together. Written goal-setting is an excellent way to crystallise your thoughts and aims for life in each area.

2. Coping mechanisms

We must shed our lives of our bad coping mechanisms and increase our good coping mechanisms. Our bad coping mechanisms include addictions, anger, negativity, jealousy and psychological symptoms. We need to clearly identify where we fall down in these areas and bring in steps that will allow us to change.

Good coping mechanisms need to be nurtured. These include time, de-clutter, positivity and humour, extracurricular activities and self-development.

Many people have very poor time-management skills and these need to be improved either at a personal level or even with the help of a counsellor or a coach. Lots of people live in clutter. They have messy offices, messy studies, messy sheds, messy houses. Mess in this area means mess in our emotions and mess in our mind. Minimise the amount of 'stuff' you have and keep your mind clear.

A positive outlook and a sense of humour is vital for a general sense of wellbeing. It is important to have activities outside of work and outside of home. Sport is an excellent form of stress management. I suggest people have regular remedial or Swedish massage, which is a wonderful form of relaxation and also excellent for body toning. You should also see every day as a self-development program.

3. Relationships

Our relationships with people—either our primary relationship or our relationship with other members of our family, our friends, our acquaintances and our work associates—is a vital part of our life. It is so important to put time and effort into all of your relationships—especially those people who will be there for the long haul.

4. Creative techniques

One of our modern-day spiritual leaders is Eckhart Tolle, who wrote the book *The Power of Now*. Tolle makes the important point that all life is this very moment. Living in the moment is vital. There are so many people who live in the past or are worried about the future and, by doing so, lose the ability to derive the maximum benefit from the present moment. Again, much lip service is given to this point, but there doesn't appear to be much action. So many people allow traumas of the past, that might've occurred for an hour or so of their life, to determine their behaviour for the next 30, 40 or 50 years.

So many people spend their time worrying about what may possibly happen in the future, but in most cases it doesn't eventuate anyhow. So many people have health fears. I have many patients in my clinic who, for 10 years, have been worried that because their father had a heart attack in his forties they are also going to do the same. When I assess them with our highly accurate screening methods I'm able to reassure them that the chance of this happening is extremely low. They've therefore spent years worrying for nothing.

How many people travel to work by the same route every day and really don't take in any of the wonderful scenery but spend their time worrying about aspects of their life that are probably not that important? How much time is spent on dislike, or at times even hatred, of another person? This certainly has no value whatsoever.

Another important creative technique is to spend half an hour every day as your own time. During this half-hour you should attempt to wind your thought processes down to nothing. I believe the best technique to do this is to use some form of meditation. I personally perform transcendental meditation every day; and even forgetting the spiritual benefits of this technique, transcendental meditation is now being shown in many clinical studies to reduce high blood pressure and coronary heart disease, and decrease hospitalisation rates. People who meditate regularly are much less likely to smoke and, surprisingly, have lower cholesterol levels.

Although I feel the world would be a better place if everyone meditated, there is no doubt that meditation is not for everybody. I have had so many people say, 'I have tried this and have failed miserably.' Try sitting in a room listening to Mozart for half an hour with your eyes closed. Water the garden for half an hour. Sit on the back porch with a glass of red looking over the view for half an hour. Just have that time with yourself every day for half an hour and, I promise you, you will derive enormous benefits. The simple practice of sitting quietly by yourself reduces your risk for heart disease and cancer by around 50 to 60 per cent.

5. Action

The points in this section have been discussed before. They not only apply to stress management, but also to all aspects of life. Unless you start to bring in steps to change, nothing will ever happen. Action, therefore, involves five components:

- **Decision:** Once you have made a decision to change an aspect of your life, this is the obvious starting point.
- **Interrupt the limiting patterns:** Find out what is stopping you from achieving your goal at the moment and work very hard on these aspects.
- **Create a new pattern.**
- **Condition the new pattern:** When anything new occurs in your life it will be unnatural for you to perform these actions. You must discipline yourself for one month and after that the new pattern will be part of your life.
- **Live the program:** Don't see any desirable goal as something you will follow for a few months. See it as a new part of your life and make sure you intend to live the way you desire.

To maintain this action, you must also follow these general steps:

(i) *Review all of your goals daily.* Keep a journal and review your goals on all aspects of your life every day.

324

(ii) *Review the plan.* It is not good enough just to have a goal; you must also have a workable plan that will allow you to achieve that goal. Review your plan every day to reinforce the steps needed to achieve the goal.

(iii) *Take small steps.* Confucius said, 'A journey of a thousand miles begins with a single step.' Perform some aspect of your goal every day; for example, if you want to learn a new language, just by learning five new words every day you will have learned a new language in about 12 months.

(iv) *Visualise your goal achievement.* Visualisation is a very powerful technique that will help you to focus.

(v) *Monitor your progress.* In your goal journal, write down how you are doing—either from a positive or a negative sense.

It has been said that the only things that are certain in life are death and taxes. I would like to add that I believe that stress is also an absolute certainty. No matter how smoothly our life appears to be going, there will always be days or weeks when some unexpected stress occurs. This can be of a minor nature or, less frequently, of a major nature.

The most important advice is to see stress as a great teacher and learning experience. Of course, it feels lousy at the time; but, I promise you, you will be a better person for it. In the words of the great Viktor Frankl: 'It is not the suffering, but the way you handle the suffering that is important.'

For any further information on Dr Ross Walker regarding subscriptions to *The Walker Health Report*, refer to the website: **www.whr.com.au**

If you would like to book Dr Ross Walker as a speaker at a conference or any corporate function, please contact:

The Fordham Company
PO Box 820
Woollahra NSW 1350
Australia

Tel: 61 2 9362 0040
Fax: 61 2 9362 0707
Email: info@thefordhamcompany.com.au
Website: www.thefordhamcompany.com.au